Copyrights

Tatiana Barrera reserves the right to be identified as author of this Work. Said right has been asserted by her in accordance with sections 77 and 78 of the Copyright, Designs and Patents Act 1988. All rights reserved. No part of this publication may be reproduced, stored in retrieval system, copied in any form or by any means, electronic, mechanical, photocopying, recording or otherwise transmitted without written permission from the author. You must not share or circulate this book in any format.

"No Milk, Please" like any other printed or electronic book, is protected by international laws of authorship and intellectual property. The copy or distribution of this document, in part or in whole, constitutes a crime.

The recipes included in the book are courtesy of different chefs from around the globe, who reserve all authorship rights and are protected by the laws mentioned before.

Aquasana LLC
401 E. Las Olas Boulevard, Suite 130-410
Fort Lauderdale, FL 33301

All rights reserved under Copyright Conventions.
Copyright ©2012 Tatiana Barrera

ISBN: 978-0615752976
ISBN: 0615752977

For ordering information, please contact
Tatiana@TatianaBarrera.com
1-(561) 318-1292

Notice

The information in this book reflects the investigations and experience of the author. It is intended to serve for educational purposes but not as medical advice, and it does not replace the advice of your health professional. The suggestions presented do not guarantee the cure or prevention of any specific health condition.

Table of Content

ABOUT THE AUTHOR

DEDICATION

INTRODUCTION

WHY DO THEY RECOMMEND US TO DRINK MILK?

WHAT ALTERNATIVES ARE THERE TO MILK?

HISTORY OF MILK CONSUMPTION

CHANGING CULTURAL PARADIGMS

HOW TO REPLACE MILK?

CALCIUM

PROTEIN

PROTECTING OUR BONE HEALTH

BREAKING PARADIGMS

NO MILK PLEASE

VEGETABLE MILKS

SOY MILK

HOW TO PREPARE VEGETABLE MILKS

HYDRATION, HYDRATION, HYDRATION

CONCLUSION

RECIPES

REFERENCES

About the Author

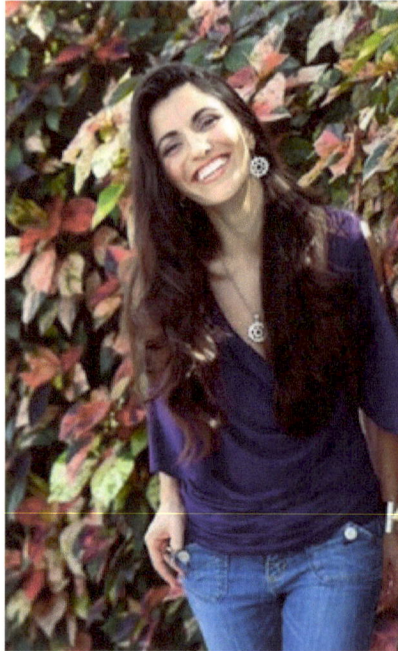

Tatiana Barrera was born and raised in Bogota, Colombia. Coming from a family of farmers, she has her best childhood memories from the countryside, enjoying nature and the animals. She remembers how one of the greatest pleasures for her father was to get up early in the morning to enjoy a full glass freshly milked. Which came from cows that spent their lives free in the open outdoors, rotating fields to allow the grass to recover after their pass. These were animals that were treated with love and respect, and allowed to save part of their milk for their calves.

There was a balance in the coexistence; the family and the animals that shared this paradise lived in harmony without abuse or mistreatments. The harvests were colorful and generous. Depending on the time of year, there was abundance of mango, bananas or oranges. Fruits and vegetables were enjoyed vine ripened, fresh and free of chemicals. Diet would vary according to the season.

But life and experience showed Tatiana that not everything works in the same way as in her father's farm. She graduated as an Industrial Engineer, and her professional career opened her eyes to how different the food industry is from those childhood memories she treasures. Food is processed and saved throughout the year, so everything is available all year round. It is no longer natural and fresh; it is different: it comes from a factory.

Her constant desire to study and learn more about the things she is passionate about, and her love for the environment, took her career through a path of growth and discovery. As a mother, her main motivation is her kids. The ability to offer them the best quality of life possible and leave them, and other children, a healthier world to live in is of primordial importance. At first, she channeled her career through ecology and environmental conservation. Later, she dedicated herself to nutrition. As Tatiana says, "We can't save the environment if we don't save ourselves at the same time."

Today, Tatiana is an author and public speaker, spreading the word of balanced nutrition and healthy lifestyle. Her experiences, the fact that she has lived in three different countries, and her constant desire to read in-between the lines and to find what lies underneath anything life puts in her path are her strongest tools. Her experience as a member of the Institute for Integrative Nutrition® - IIN® - has allowed her to broaden her vision about nutrition and to develop the concept of what she calls an Alkaline Lifestyle. A lifestyle of balance. A balance inside our body, in our relationships, and with the environment. In her website (www.TatianaBarrera.com) she affirms:

When I try to define an Alkaline Lifestyle, a quote from John Lennon comes to mind: "When I was 5 years old, my mother always told me that Happiness was the key to Life. When I went to school, they asked me what I wanted to be when I grew up. I wrote down 'Happy'. They told me I didn't understand the assignment, and I told them they didn't understand Life." To attain that happiness in our day to day, life has taught me that several things need to be in balance; our body, soul, heart and surroundings. That balance equals an Alkaline Lifestyle.

Dedication

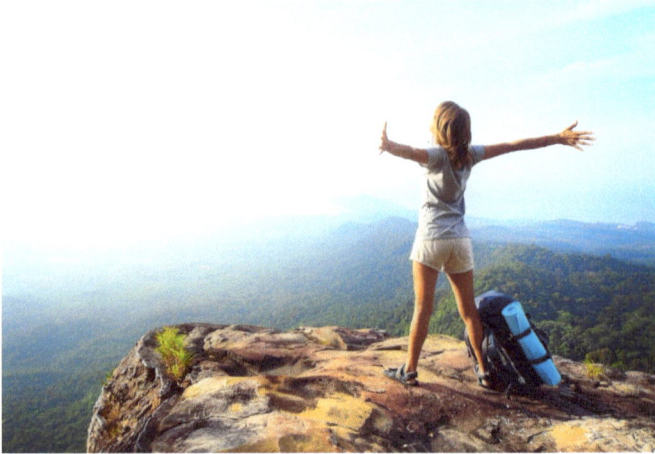

Words are not enough to thank God, life and every single person that has been part of this project in one way or another.

Thanks to my children, my inspiration, my motivation, my reason for being. Dreams do come true. We all deserve to be healthy and happy. That is why we came to this world. Never stop smiling and being happy. This book, as well as all my work and efforts are for you and because of you.

To my parents, my sister and my brother, I am ever thankful. I have you in my heart at every second and feel your presence and support embracing me all along. Thanks for believing in me. Thanks for the past, the present, and the future. I am who I am thanks to you.

To Marie Baccini, Paula Labbad-Smith and Silvia Labbad, I am eternally grateful. Not only for sharing your incredible culinary talents, but above all, for being friends, family, and adding the ingredients of laughter and love to every recipe and in every stage of this process.

Special thanks to the following chefs for their generosity in sharing their recipes with us:

Chef Elena Dal Forno, in Treviso, Italy http://Facebook.com/RawVeganChefElena
Mel with Balance pH Diet http://Balance-ph-diet.com
Chef Barry Kraemer, http://ChefKraemer.com
David Choi, Buddhist vegetarian chef dedicated to collaborating with his recipes and lessons to change the lifestyle of society.
Chef Erik Mathes, http://www.linkedin.com/in/erikmathes

Thanks to you too - to each of you reading these lines - for allowing me inside your home to share with you my ideas. I sincerely hope to be able to contribute to your, and your family's health.

Introduction

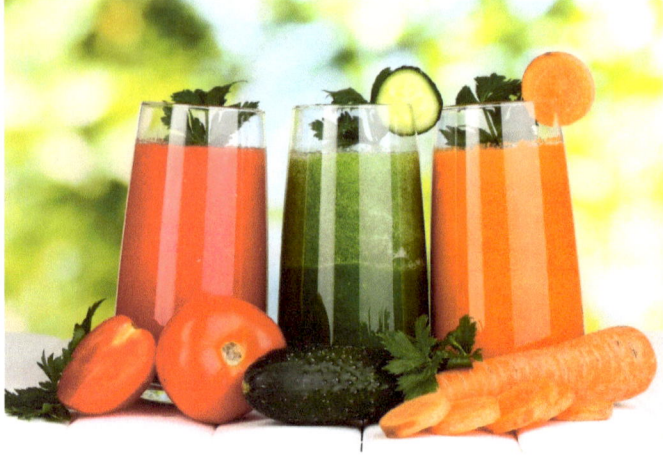

More and more people are turning away from the consumption of milk and dairy products. Some do it because of problems with lactose. Others do it because of problems with casein, which constitutes between 85% and 90% of milk protein[1]. Some others do it in search of healthier alternatives in their diet, or because they reject the strong environmental impact that this industry represents - both with its emission of waste liquids, solids and gases (greenhouse effect), and the consumption of water and other elements.[2,3,4,5]

Regardless of personal motives, it is a fact that milk is no longer the unquestioned constant in a healthy diet. The intention of this book is not to focus on the disadvantages of drinking milk. My aim is rather to share some information that most people ignore or are simply unaware of. You will then assess the nutritional alternatives you have available to replace the consumption of dairy in your diet, thus introducing healthier options for your menu.

Remember that just as personality, emotional needs and levels of physical activity are unique for each person. So is diet. The main problem with modern diets is the fact that they approach food with a "one size fits all" attitude. The truth is that no diet is perfect for everyone. We are different and it is these differences that we need to identify in order to give our body the best nutrition possible.

       As Joshua Rosenthal[6] states, "it is important to learn to listen to our bodies". The way we feel after eating a certain food is the language that our body uses to tell if it's a food that contributes to your health or if it makes you vulnerable to imbalance.

Why do they recommend us to drink milk?

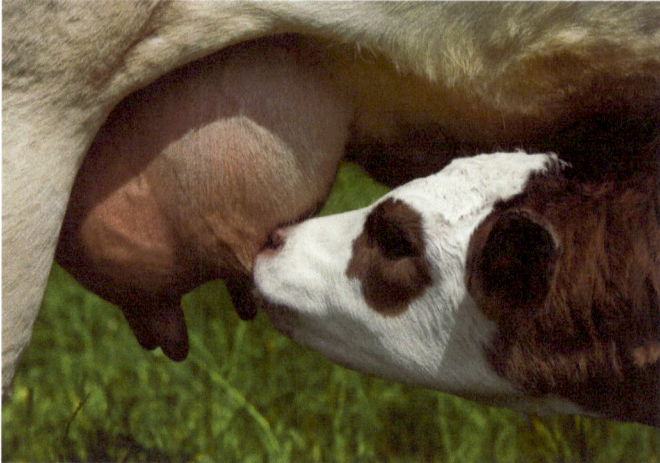

Milk has been over-praised in our Western culture. A constant, long unquestioned part of a balanced diet. But if we look at this issue a little closer, we discover that milk contains nutrients that are also present in various other foods. I dare to say that if we analyze them one by one, we can find natural sources where that nutrient is in a purer form that can be more easily assimilated by our body.

The following properties are attributed to milk and dairy products:

Calcium:

Calcium is an important mineral for the health of our bones and teeth. It helps maintain muscle mass, and plays an important role in blood clotting, in nervous system function, in certain hormonal processes, in regulating our muscle functions, and in maintaining pH balanced at a cellular level. But we cannot forget that even though we have more calcium than other minerals in the body, calcium is one of more than 12 minerals necessary for healthy functioning and development of the same. In fact, when we consume calcium together with magnesium, for example, the body can absorb it better and benefits from it more effectively. So calcium should be thought of as part of an equation rather than a "one man show".

Protein:

Proteins are responsible for building and repairing our muscle tissue along with other tissues in the body, as well as synthesizing enzymes and strengthening the immune system. The first of these functions is potentiated in periods of high growth of our body, which is from when we are babies until we finish our development at the age of 18-20. As the growth rate slows, our need to consume proteins also decreases. Its other functions do persist throughout our lives though.

But when it comes to proteins, we face a conceptual problem: how much protein does the human body really need to stay healthy? In Western cultures we consume much more protein than our body actually needs. Recommendations vary greatly; they are confusing and often exaggerated. It is important to remember that, just as a low intake of protein is harmful to health, so is the over consumption of it.

The key is being able to maintain a balance, keeping in mind that all extremes are bad. Going back to the actual definition of protein, perhaps the first thing that comes to mind when you think of protein is "meat" or other animal products such as milk or eggs. Well, reality turns out not to be as simple. There are many types of proteins, thousands in fact, in both animals and plants. And they all have one thing in common: they are composed of amino acids. Proteins are then essentially just a chain of amino acids joined to form a larger structure.

Now, if we start from the premise that amino acids are what make up a protein, we can understand that these building blocks are what our body really needs to form the different protein it requires. In fact, our body cannot benefit from the protein itself when consumed. As part of the digestive process, the organism needs to break it into amino acids so that they can travel to our cells, then join with other amino acids and form the different proteins that specific parts of our system need. We will talk about the various available sources of these amino acids further in the book.

Potassium, phosphorus, vitamins A, B2, B12, D and niacin:

All these essential elements are part of the list of benefits attributed to dairy products. But again, all of them can be found more abundantly and easier to be absorbed in other foods; we will review those in later chapters.

What alternatives are there to milk?

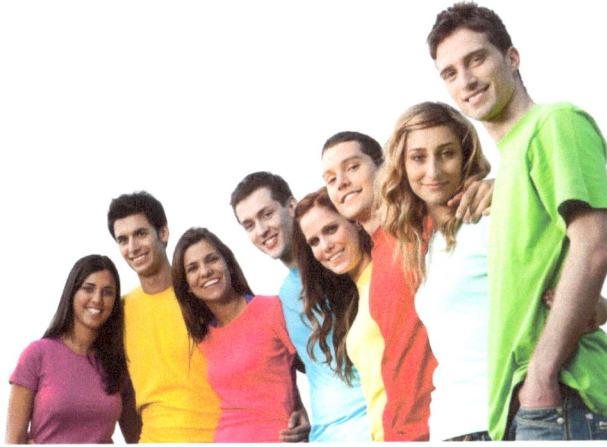

In speaking about replacing milk in our diet, there are two things that we are replacing. First is the milk as a source of nutrients. Second is milk as a concept, or as part of what we have been taught that it is a balanced diet. We will go deeper into the nutritional aspect in a moment. Now let's take a look at the intangible side of milk, that cultural aspect that is also being reassessed when thinking of a dairy free diet.

How can something that has always been said to be healthy be actually bad for us?

Let's keep in mind that each of us is different, and what is good for one person may be harmful to another. This is the main message to remember. Education is power, and learning about the different alternatives of nutritional sources available to us is the key to achieving balance and living a healthy life. Once this information is presented to us, we must analyze it from our unique situation, and be aware of how your body reacts to one type of food or another.

In nutrition there are no generalizations, in fact those can actually be extremely dangerous. We are unique beings and so are our bodies. That said, I invite you to take the information in this book, and any other source of nutritional counseling you find available, as a tool to increase your knowledge, but not as a dogma or a law.

It is also worth to note that, even if you decide to completely abolish milk from your diet, it will still be part of the eating habits of others and of our cultural environment, then it is likely that it will still be present at family and friends' gatherings. Given this, I quote again an idea from Joshua Rosenthal, who speaks of the primary food (our relationships) as food for the soul, being crucial to our good health. When these situations arise, and you are offered a dairy based dinner, for example, remember that your relationship with the host should be most important to you at the time. Face the dilemma with love and respect, not judgment or rejection. Allow yourself the opportunity to make an exception maybe, and eat the lasagna with cheese, or balance your plate in the way you consider healthiest without making your host feel like you reject their food or judge their preferences. This will remove the pressure from the environment and will allow you and others to enjoy the gathering better. Remember, if 70% of everything you eat responds to your idea of a healthy diet, there is room in that other 30% to have a little flexibility.

To better understand the cultural aspect of milk dependence, let's start by reviewing the history of the consumption of milk by humans. When did we begin to drink milk? Is today's milk the same as what our ancestors drank?

When we realize the great changes that this food has undergone through history, we can demystify its importance and reevaluate our idea of milk as a suitable source of nutrition.

History of Milk Consumption

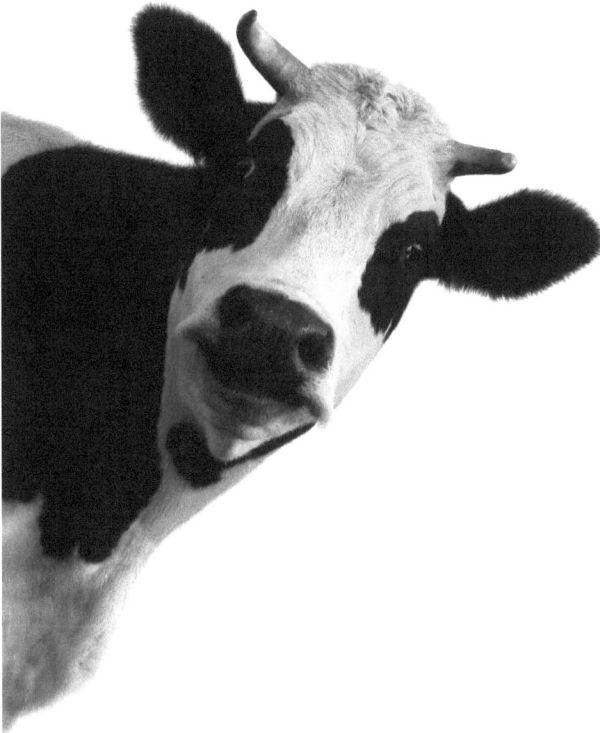

The consumption of milk by humans dates back some ~7,500 years. At the time, humans were transitioning from being nomadic, to settling as farmers. We are talking specifically about the population in the region between the Balkans and Central Europe. As they began to make their settlements, these prehistoric ancestors began to domesticate animals. Sheep were first to be domesticated and then followed other animals such as aurochs - ancestor, now extinct of the cow.[7,8,9] Cheese consumption dates back to about the same period.[76,77]

For these early farmers to be able to digest milk in adulthood a number of genetic changes had to take place. As mammals once we overcome infancy, we lose the ability to produce lactase: the enzyme needed to digest milk. Before these Neolithic farmers became able to produce this enzyme in adulthood, it took between 1,000 and 2,000 years[7] and a series of evolutionary processes. In fact, only part of the population from this region was really able to produce lactase into adulthood. For those who did - specifically in northern regions- this fact is explained as a genetic adaptation to outweigh the lack of sun: a main source of vitamin D, needed to absorb calcium.

Over time, other farmer cultures began to also develop the ability to drink milk, but it was never more than a minority who managed to adapt to digest it without it constituting a burden on their digestion or a problem for their health. Today, a high percentage of adults worldwide do not produce this enzyme (lactase) and are therefore unable to digest lactose.

The evolutionary step to achieve the digestion of milk occurred almost simultaneously in Europe and parts of Asia and Africa. For the Native American population, on the other hand, it was not until the sixteenth century [7] that livestock was first introduced. This means that this part of American ancestry did not participate in the evolutionary adaptation described.

However, milk consumption became widespread and began to be embraced in various cultures, without scientific awareness of its health effects. Even today, many suffer the consequences of this, without even knowing it. Experts in the field have found that problems such as abdominal pain, asthma, sinusitis, iron deficiencies, cardiovascular disease, osteoporosis, acne, cataracts, arthritis and even cancer, may be related to dairy consumption.[10,11,12] Unfortunately, this information is not available to everyone, and many of those who suffer from such ailments ignore their possible relationship with dairy.

There's a parallel issue and it is the change in the quality of the milk we consume. It is not the same to talk about the raw milk the first farmers in the Balkans had access to, than to talk about the homogenized pasteurized milk we consume in the present.

In the nineteenth century, the French chemist and biologist Louis Pasteur discovered the relationship between certain diseases and germs from foods like milk. Pasteur invented the pasteurization process in order to kill these microorganisms. And while it is true that this process eliminated the risk of many infectious diseases, it also alters the nutritional composition of the milk, reducing its vitamin C content, killing beneficial bacteria, and exposing us to a new range of possible problems.[13,14,15]

In 1899, Auguste Gaulin invents the process of homogenization, in which the milk is passed under pressure through microscopic nozzles. This process reduces fat globules to a minimum so that milk doesn't "separate". The process not only changes the color of milk and natural property of "separating", but it also makes certain enzymes become so small, that they are now able to go through the intestinal lining into the bloodstream. These enzymes produce an imbalance that can compromise the integrity of our arterial walls by potentially lacerating them. So, to protect itself, the body increases its production of cholesterol, accumulating it on the walls of veins and arteries.[16,17,18] In other words, the process of homogenization of milk can be highly related to the "epidemic" of cardiovascular disease we are experiencing today.

The pasteurization, and later the homogenization processes, gave rise to mass commercialization of milk. Years ago, this product was sold in glass bottles and was distributed from house to house on a daily basis by a milkman. But around 1950, comes a rapid industrialization and the food system begins one of the most radical changes in the history of mankind. In fact, it is said that our eating habits have changed more in the last 100 years than they did in the previous 10,000.[19,20]

If we think of the hundreds of years of evolutionary process that took our ancestors to achieve the ability to digest milk, then it should not be a surprise to see that with such rapid change in our diet over the past decades, we are exposing our bodies to foods for which we are not ready. This could support the explanation of the number of degenerative diseases, cancers, and cardiovascular problems we are seeing in today's society.

The food industry has dramatically changed in the last 50 years, and needless to say, the dairy sector is no exception.[21,22,23] Today, a dairy cow in the United States produces more than twice the amount of milk produced by her ancestors in the 1950's.[24,25] This excessive production brings several consequences. It not only shortens the life expectancy of the animal to almost a quarter of its longevity under natural conditions, but it can also carry along health problems with it.[26] Many of these cows develop mastitis - a localized infection in the udder - and / or lacerations because of the industrialized milking. These expose the milk to becoming contaminated with blood, pus and secretions derived from said conditions.[27,28,29]. Cows also develop other ailments caused by the abnormal size of their udders; which makes it hard for them to walk, and generates pelvic and spinal problems. We're talking about potentially diseased animals that are overfed (mainly with corn, not grass) to a degree of obesity, that have little, or no physical activity, and receive minimal sun exposure. The current livestock is far from that picturesque setting where animals lived in the open outdoors and fed on grass. Today the dairy cattle is raised and treated in a radically different fashion than before. The grass, their natural food, was slowly replaced by corn and other supplements: less expensive alternatives that made the cows fatter faster and that accelerated their milk production. Cattle stopped walking free in the sun, and began to grow up in overcrowded facilities, under conditions that are very different from what would be considered as natural. As if this was not enough, in order to boost their growth, and to counteract the problems that cows developed by their sedentary lives, they are undergoing hormone and antibiotics treatments that bring along a whole new range of threats to our health.

We are not talking about the same milk anymore.

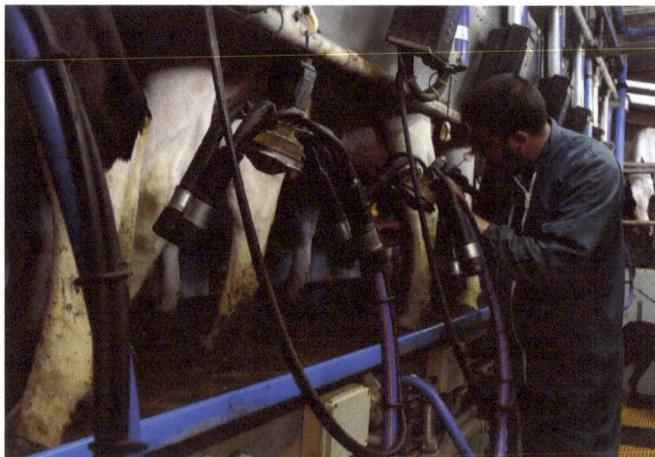

Changing cultural paradigms

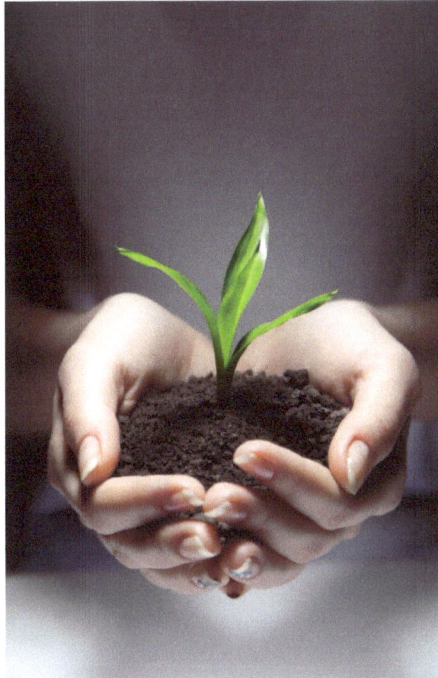

We are all different, and therefore there is no mold in which every one of us would fit. Each of us is not only unique, but also in constant evolution. Change is life; change is being reborn to new ideas and possibilities. Let us celebrate these differences and escape some of those preconceived or inculcated ideas.

For people whose ancestry comes from Scandinavian regions, for example, milk has always been part of the diet and culture, and their bodies evolved to accept it into the diet. But as we saw earlier, this adaptation was given specifically to accept raw milk from animals feeding on grass and sun; not pasteurized and homogenized milk from animals raised with supplements, in an industrial environment.

For those who enjoy the consumption of milk or its derivatives - and are not interested or willing to eliminate them from their diet - the quality of these products must become priority. Although it is slowly regaining popularity, raw milk is difficult to find, and may present in itself, a number of other potential health risks. But if that is not an option, knowing the origin and quality of the dairy consumed, and choosing organic milk from animals that have been treated fairly and properly can make a big difference.

As I mentioned before, and it is worth repeating, information is power. There are times when the understanding of certain things can change our minds - or reaffirm ideas intuitively presaged - and therefore re-adjust the way we think and act. This is the change experienced by many when they investigate deeper into the milk ordeal. But we have a strong impediment in achieving such change at a social level, and this obstacle is the mass marketing of milk. Keep in mind that the dairy industry is one of the largest and wealthiest sectors of our economy, and thus has a strong influence in both politics and media.

Therefore, this must be a personal process, or small-scale adaptation of our customs. And for those who are considering reducing or eliminating dairy products from your diet, I can say from personal experience - and the experience of people with whom I have had the pleasure of working - that this change is much easier than it may at first appear. We have so many delicious and healthy alternatives, that the process is, honestly, more a pleasure than a chore.

To me, what is happening with the marketing of milk is a situation similar to what happened between the 20s and 50s with the cigarette industry. If you remember, at that time there were television commercials where doctors, athletes, and even Santa Claus would promote smoking as a healthy way to relieve stress and feel better. This was part of the culture, accepted and promoted in the daily life of society.[30] If they knew of the detrimental effect of cigarettes on health, no one would talk about it.

The lesson is then to not accept what is presented to us as an absolute truth. We are constantly bombarded with information from different media. Take it, analyze it, confirm it with other sources you trust, and keep only what you deem valuable, discarding the rest.

How to replace milk?

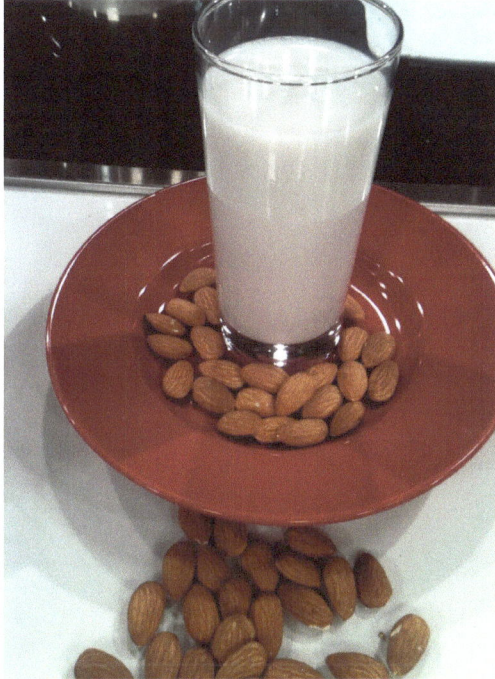

Lets look now into practical solutions to the issue in question. Vegetable alternatives exist that can be used much like a traditional milk. The vegetable milks are basically beverages derived from grains, legumes, nuts and seeds that are a parallel option or substitute the consumption of animal milks.

There are broad varieties of plant milks that are commercially available, or that can be easily prepared at home. Each of them offers a different taste and nutritional content, presenting a wide range to choose from. In general, most of these substitutes to cow's milk can be considered healthier than the same, because they have a much lower content of saturated fats and cholesterol.

Milks of almond, flax, coconut, hemp, rice... the alternatives are numerous. The vegetable milks can be used in many ways and the variety of flavors allows us to play with them and develop new and delicious recipes. The almond, hazelnut, walnut or oat milks are ideal for the preparation of cakes, and many desserts. The latter has a much milder flavor, thus not altering the taste of the recipe. Each of the nut milks has its own flavor, which can be a delicious way to vary your creations.

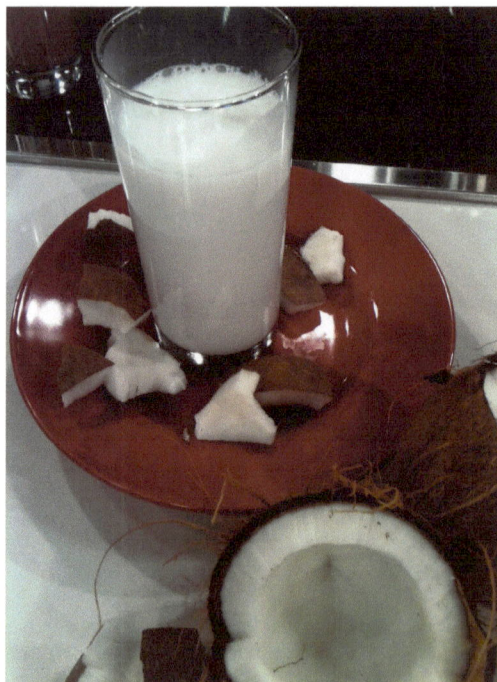

The vegetable milks are not only very healthy and tasty, but can also be very economical when we prepare them ourselves. We will talk about how to make them at home later in the book. For now, lets concentrate on considering their nutritional qualities, and talk about the nutrients that we need to replace after eliminating cow's milk from our diet.

Our organism has certain basic nutritional requirements to stay healthy. These include calcium and protein - main benefits attributed to milk. Below, I will present some alternative sources of these nutrients for people who have a diet free of dairy.

Calcium

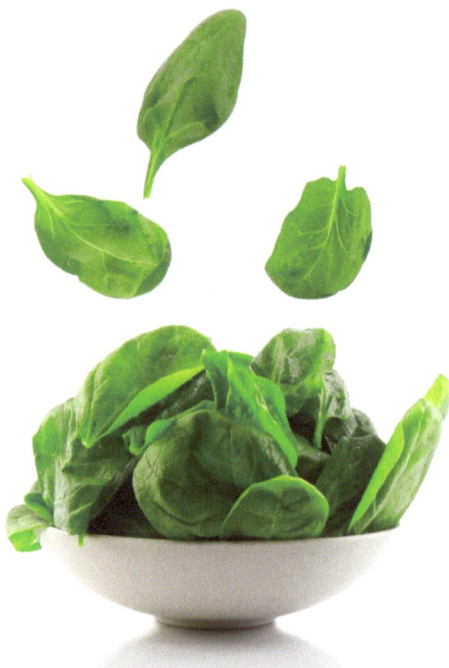

Most of the calcium in our body resides in the bones and teeth, and is responsible for maintaining their strength and consistency. A smaller percentage of this mineral in the organism travels through the bloodstream and is also found in the soft tissues, being responsible for proper muscle contraction, nerve connectivity and circulation. Therefore, eating a diet rich in calcium is imperative to stay healthy.

But our society has over-praised calcium, ignoring the fact that this is not the only important mineral in our body. When we have an excess of calcium in the body but not enough magnesium, phosphorus, boron, copper, manganese and zinc, we increase our risk of bone problems.[6] The key, as always, is to aim for balance, too much of one thing and too little of another can open the door to problems and diseases.

Although milk is recognized as one of the best sources of calcium available, it is fundamental to note that one thing is to talk about the calcium content in a certain food, and another, is the level of absorption of this nutrient once it enters our system. For example, a maximum of 32% of the total calcium in cow milk is absorbable by the organism[31]. Now, if there is some degree of intolerance in the body, which is the case in a great percentage of the population, the body is forced to use its mineral reserves to aid in digestion, and the net effect is that of nutritional drainage instead of contribution.

Looking now at the counterpart, calcium present in plant sources, offers a higher level of absorption by the body. These are just a few examples of it:

Vegetable	Percentage of Calcium absorption[31]
Broccoli	53%
Brussels sprouts	64%
Mustard Greens	64%
Kale	40 to 59%

The consumption of these foods also provides an **alkalizing** effect on the cellular level. This means it helps set the minerals in the bones, and keep our reserves of calcium and other minerals in the body. It also means it helps to stabilize the pH of our tissues and bloodstream. A balance that allows us to prevent disease, stay healthy, and energized. We use the term "alkalizing"[78] to describe foods that benefit the pH balance in the organism, as the body's natural pH is slightly alkaline.

Another benefit of consuming calcium in the form of green vegetables is that it comes accompanied with magnesium, an important mineral that further helps to fix calcium, and other minerals.

The above are just some examples of vegetables rich in highly absorbable calcium, but we can also add to this list: spinach, watercress, oranges, almonds, seaweed, sesame seeds, parsley and beans, among others.

Regarding the content of calcium, in terms of percentages, said plant sources constitute better alternatives to cow milk. For example, for each unit of calcium contained in milk, here is the content of calcium in other foods[32]:

Almonds Kale Watercress Parsley	Contains 2 units
Spinach	Contains 2.5 units
Sesame seeds	Contain 5 units!

Almonds, for example, are rich in calcium, vitamin E, phosphorus, iron and magnesium. Being a great source of protein, they are also good sources of zinc, selenium, copper and niacin - important minerals for our health.

Consuming enough calcium should not be a problem even if you never eat a dairy product again, considering the wide variety of foods rich in it. The key is to understand which are the best sources of this mineral and make sure to include them in your diet. Check with your health care professional to determine your specific requirements of calcium.

It is also important to note that it is not just what we do to consume calcium from the diet, but also what we do to conserve calcium we already have in our body. Our lifestyle plays an important roll here. Here are some tips you can implement:

No smoking or being exposed to secondhand smoke. The body uses its mineral reserves to counteract the harmful effects of smoking, which has acidifying consequences. In order to do so, calcium and other minerals need to be drained from our system, which makes us more vulnerable to disease and premature aging.
Sun bathing. The sun is a natural source of life and vitamin D. Moderate sun exposure helps us fix the calcium we consume.
Exercise. Physical activity and exercise, in combination with a balanced

diet, promote healthy joints and improve bone density, maintaining adequate reserves of calcium in the bones.

Before wrapping up the subject of calcium, I want to touch on the controversial issue of calcium supplements. Although there is a place for these in the treatment of specific conditions, the consumption of calcium supplements and other isolated supplements has become widespread in our society to a point that it is no longer healthy. Our body is made to absorb the nutrients in their original form. Natural foods contain thousands of nutrients in small quantities that interact with each other producing a synergy that potentiates them and benefits our health. When we consume one or a few of these nutrients, in mega-doses, we risk putting your organism in a position that compromises its normal functioning. Or we may just be wasting our money, as most of these supplements go through our system and are expelled from it without the body being able to benefit from them.

Further problems with calcium supplements have been unveiled too. Recently, much controversy has been generated about these, since their consumption has been associated with an increased incidence of heart attacks.[33,34,35] Additionally, if we look at worldwide tendencies, countries that invest the most money in vitamins and calcium supplements specifically are those with the highest incidence of osteoporosis.

Protein

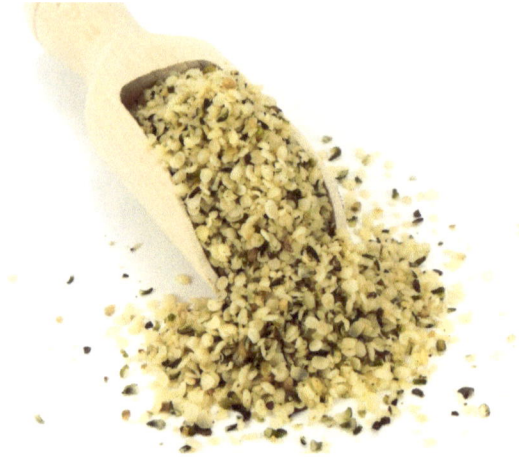

Proteins, macromolecules made up of a chain of amino acids, are vital to our health, and constitute approximately 15% to 20% of the human body. Protein requirements vary throughout life, we need greater amounts of them during the growing years, or when the body is recovering from specific situations such as burns or big losses of blood, among others.

Our body produces a large variety of proteins (remember: chain amino acids) to meet its different needs, from building new cellular structures and regulating the function of organs and tissues, to transporting nutrients and oxygen through its system. They carry, for example, collagen to the connective tissues, hair and nails and play an important role in our enzymatic and hormonal functions.

When we consume proteins, the body breaks them down and creates what we could call an amino acid pool, from which it will supply itself of the specific ones it needs for making up the different new proteins.

Amino acids are chemical compounds containing carbon, hydrogen, oxygen and nitrogen. There are two types of them, essential and non-essential.

There are nine essential amino acids, and they need to be consumed through food since our body is unable to produce them on its own. And the non-essential, are those that the body can synthesize from others already present in its system.

I took the time to explain this issue in some detail, at the risk of boring my readers with a biochemistry class, but I did it with a very clear motive in mind. Once we understand the basic concept of the formation of proteins, we can be in better position to make better decisions about our food; decisions that will be beneficial to our health and that won't put us at risk of deficiencies or problems.

With that said, there are two ways to consume protein or amino acids in our diet. These are the complete and the incomplete proteins. The complete proteins contain all 9 of the essential amino acids. Most of these sources of complete protein are of animal origin. Incomplete proteins are foods that lack one or more of the essential amino acids. But the word "incomplete" should in no way have a negative connotation, and that's what I want to emphasize, because we can combine "incomplete" foods to complement each other, and add up to the 9 essential amino acids our bodies need. For example, if we combine certain vegetables with whole grains, we build the net protein unit, which accounts for a complete protein source.

Lets look into which foods are good sources of protein.

Among the animal sources, we have the different meats, poultry, fish, dairy and eggs. But just as we analyzed how the dairy industry has become so industrialized, something very similar has happened with the livestock, poultry and fish industries. For this reason, if you decide to consume animal products, it is essential to know their origin and quality. The following can be considered good sources of animal protein:

Cow meat, provided it comes from cattle that has been bred and fed in free grazing, with a chance to exercise their muscles and take sun. This is very different from eating meat that comes from cattle that has been raised with grains, injected with hormones and antibiotics, or kept in intensive overcrowding.[36]
Organic chicken. Similarly, when the chicken has been raised naturally, outdoors and with adequate food, they may constitute a good source of lean protein. Eggs, as well, must come from animals raised organically; otherwise

they may have many more threats to our health, than potential benefits. Early in the book, when talking about the dairy industry, I drew a picture of the livestock sector in general. In my opinion, the poultry farming has undergone the same - or worse - evolution. We will not go into the details now, but the next time you go to the supermarket, look at the size of the chicken breasts they sell. I invite to ask yourself... How can a normal chicken carry so much weight? The sad truth is that most of them can't ... this is the result of an abuse in the production process in spite of the animal's health. Now, please think about the consequences for these animals and how they will reflect in your health.[37]

Wild fish. The term "wild" refers to animals that were born and raised in their natural habitat. Be it salmon, tuna or other fish variety, it should come from wild origin rather than a farmed environment, since the latter develop high levels of toxicity and heavy metals in certain instances. Not all fish is healthy; only wild fish are able to reach the desired levels of Omega-3 and can be a source of balanced nutrition.[38,39,40,41]

Before listing the sources of vegetable protein, I want to review some of the advantages they may represent to our health:

Vegetable protein sources are also rich in minerals, which allows them to be less acidifying to the blood and instead, provide us the health benefit of helping balance the natural pH of the cells.

Because of its composition, with fewer purines and more fiber, they are easier to digest, their wastes are disposed from our body faster and easier, and this reduces the risk of accumulation of uric acid, which causes gout and other health problems.

They have less fat, saturated fat and cholesterol and have a better caloric balance than animal protein sources. Benefits that are highly desirable for keeping our cardiovascular health and a healthy weight.

With the above information in mind, lets look at some examples of plant sources of protein:

Green vegetables. The dark green color of certain plants is a good sign of their high content of minerals, chlorophyll and amino acids. Kale, spinach, peas, green beans and broccoli, among others, are excellent sources of protein.

Hemp seeds. Many people mistakenly attributed a bad reputation to hemp seeds because of its remote connection to marijuana. But this reasoning cannot be further from truth. Hemp, in fact, has the opposite effect of its cousin. So even though they belong to the same family of plants, their characteristics, effects, and even their appearance, are radically different. The hemp seed is considered, by many experts, as one of the most complete sources of nutrition in nature. It is delicious and easy to consume, sprinkling it on salads, soups, or bread, or mixing it in juices and smoothies. Excellent carrier of Omega-3 and protein, containing all 9 essential amino acids. It is also a good source of minerals such as magnesium, iron and manganese, as well as vitamins and enzymes. They are also free of sugars, starches and saturated fat.[42,43,44,45] Thanks to its growing demand, it is becoming easier to find at health food stores and even supermarkets. Ask for it, when store owners see that there is interest in a particular product, even if they do not have it available at the time, they will start looking into carrying it to respond to their customers' request.

Quinoa. Quinoa is an ancient food, considered sacred by the Incas. Quinoa is a seed, but because of the way it is consumed, it is more widely known as a grain. Gluten-free, rich in minerals like iron, magnesium and manganese, and vitamin B2, enzymes and antioxidants. Contains all 9 essential amino acids in abundant quantities, making it an excellent nutritional source. It can be eaten hot, ideal to replace rice or other simple carbohydrates in our diet, or cold, mixed into your salads.[46,47,48,49]

Avocado. This fruit contains twice as much protein as other vegetables, and is a source of the 9 essential amino acids plus Omega-3. Avocados are low in cholesterol and sodium, high in fiber, vitamin C, K and folate[50] (the latter occurs naturally in certain foods, folic acid is the synthetic form). Because of their excellent nutritional content, avocados not only help rebuild muscles and tissues, but they also help strengthen the immune system to prevent disease.

Lentils and other legumes. Perhaps one of the most economical sources of protein available in the market; lentils provide excellent nutritional content. These, as well as chickpeas, beans and alfalfa, contain amino acids and minerals, which together produce a synergistic effect that is very beneficial for our health.[51,52] These can be prepared in different ways: cooking them directly or allowing them to germinate and then eat their sprouts, which potentiates their nutritional value.

Whole Grains. The different varieties of whole grains are also rich in protein and nutrients. Although their carbohydrate content is relatively higher, remember that the fact that they are "whole", makes them a good and healthy source of energy, accompanied by a high-fiber and minerals like magnesium and selenium plus folate (folic acid).[53,54,55]

Almonds and their derivatives (such as almond butter and almond milk). Rich in nutrients, as previously mentioned, with a high amino acid content - which makes them a good source of protein - they also provide us with riboflavin, magnesium, manganese and vitamin E.[56]

Seaweed. Also known as sea vegetables, although relatively new in our western culture, these foods have been part of the staple diet in Asia since ancient times. They have a high nutritional content, and produce an alkalizing effect in the body (helping to preserve the mineral reserves), which represents a number of additional benefits to our health. Sea vegetables have vitamin and mineral contents much higher than land plants, besides being a good source of protein and fiber. [57,58]

I hope this chapter has been able to create a broader picture of food that can be eaten as a good source of dietary protein. I invite you to experiment and try with the different options presented to enjoy greater food variety. As much as possible, aim to make the transition be gradual, allowing your body to adjust to the new habits you are acquiring.

Remember that a professional in the field should supervise any radical change in your diet, in order to ensure that you are meeting the needs of each specific nutrient. My intention with this book is not to present a food or diet plan, rather, my goal is to share important information that most of us don't know. There are countless options and alternatives that meet the preferences and needs of each person and I hope that the information presented here, is able to help you find the ideal way of eating according to your own principles and requirements.

Protecting our bone health

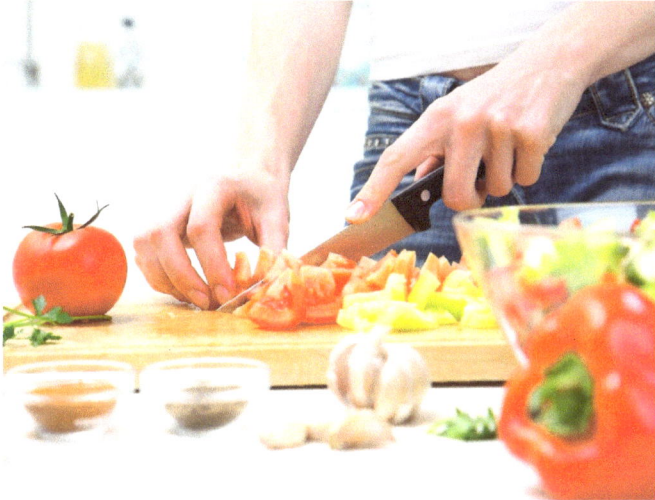

With age many people start to develop osteoporosis. This complicated word means a systemic loss in the density of our bones. The loss of density, or in other words, the relative loss of bone minerals, has several health effects, including making us vulnerable to bone fractures.

Unfortunately, most of the available information about this matter comes from the pharmaceutical industry - whose main interest is not to educate us about this or other illnesses, or help prevent them, but rather to sell us drugs and supplements that translate into revenue for them[59]. The rest of the information we receive, comes from the dairy industry, which uses every resource to position milk as the only way to maintain bone health and prevent osteoporosis.

With no intention of contradicting the advice of your doctor, I would like to explain the causes of this condition, and recommend some things that can help prevent it.

Keep in mind that our body is a unit. That every part of it operates in an orchestrated way with the rest of the organism. Thus, one cannot speak of the health of our bones without mentioning the health of our body in general. The body is a complex system that controls all functions, from the simplest, at a cellular level, to the most complex. Several parameters must be kept in balance so that the body is healthy and can regenerate and heal itself. Out of all of these parameters, perhaps the most important is the pH. In order for all biological processes - that are constantly happening in our body – to take place properly, the body must maintain its pH balanced. The pH of our blood is slightly alkaline, and has a very small range in which it can fluctuate. If you were to break out of this range, our body would cease to function, and would suffer enormous damage and even death.

One of the main challenges posed by our modern diet is the fact that it is extremely acidic. As part of our modern lifestyle, we consume too much sugar, caffeine, alcohol, processed foods and carbonated drinks. We have also become used to taking medicines as part of everyday life and not - as it should be – as an extreme measure in a specific situation. All these factors contribute to the acidification of our body.

When we eat more alkaline foods[78] than acidic foods, their alkalizing effect counteracts the negative influence of the later; allowing the organism to achieve the balance we need. But when most of our diet is made up of acidifying foods, then our body needs to use other methods to keep its pH balanced. The main method used by the organism for this purpose is to use minerals from its reserves to re-alkalize itself. What is the main reservoir of minerals in our body? Bones! So it is not surprising that, after years and years of draining minerals from the bones to counteract the effects of our diet, the density of these is diminished and affected.

Animal protein and dairy are considered specifically acidifying to our bodies, and the industrial processes through which modern milk goes through, makes it even more so. Unless we are talking about raw milk, and people with the ability to digest, I believe that it is extremely dangerous and irresponsible to market milk and dairy products as the best way to prevent osteoporosis, when in fact; they can be one of the main causes of this condition.

The question is then, how to prevent osteoporosis and other problems associated with acidosis?

Many experts agree that each disease should not be seen as a separate condition, but rather, as symptoms of an imbalance in the body.[60] This imbalance affects our metabolism, which shows in different ways. It drains our reservoirs of calcium, prevents reconstruction and repair of cells, accelerates the aging process and gives space to cell mutations to happen or to the development of diseases. If we understand in this way, we need not do a thing to prevent one disease and another to prevent the next one. What we must do, in order to lower our risk of disease, is try to keep that balance.

Several factors influence our ability to maintain balance in our body. Our lifestyle, our emotions and relationships, the environment around us, and our diet are important aspects to consider when it comes to our health.

Ideally we should strive for 70% to 80% of our diet to be alkaline foods. These foods are rich in minerals that benefit our pH balance. Overall, we can consider a food to be alkalizing if it comes from the earth. By this I mean, vegetables, grains, seeds and fruits. The counterpart, acidifying foods are those that tend to lower our pH level. Sugar, caffeine, animal protein, processed foods and medicines in general are considered acidifying. Talking about medicines, although there is an important place for them in specific situations, we must avoid turning them into part of our lifestyle as, unfortunately, it is currently happening in our society.

The concept of alkalinity, basically relates to the circulating oxygen in our blood. Having an alkaline balance means having more oxygen circulating through the body. When our system starts to acidify, we start to have less oxygen reaching our cells. This condition is associated with problems such as fatigue, insomnia, weight gain, mucus, depression and other illnesses. Diseases, including cancer, thrive in an acidic environment. When the body maintains an alkaline pH, it is more difficult for these diseases to occur, and if they start to appear, the body is in a better position to combat them and prevent them from becoming major problems.

To promote alkalinity, it is advisable to keep a diet rich in nutrients, antioxidants, minerals and amino acids that provide the body the tools for proper functioning, and promote the balance of which we spoke. This does not mean you should become a vegetarian (if you are not willing to), or change your diet dramatically. When most of your diet consists of alkalizing foods, 20% to 30% can be composed of acidic foods without having to compromise the body's normal functioning.

Food is a source of energy and life, but it is not the only one. I would say that it actually falls in second place of importance after maintaining positive relationships and emotions in our lives. Love, peace, joy and laughter are all emotions that produce chemical reactions at the level of our neurons. These emotions promote cell regeneration and alkaline balance. That feeling of tranquility and belonging, of connection with others and with the environment around us, is a source of health. And the other side of the coin is also true, stress, anger, resentment and depression promote acidosis in our system and prevent the body to regenerate and heal normally.

Another important recommendation for body, soul and mind health is physical activity and outdoor time. Movement and exercise, as well as sun exposure, increase the ability of our body to stay in balance and to combat disease and decay, while at the same time promoting positive feelings, and a sense of connection.

This chapter sought to discuss the health of our bones, but as we saw, it is impossible to talk about the health of a body part without considering the overall health of the organism. So the next time someone approaches you saying that not drinking milk puts you at risk for osteoporosis, you already know what to answer. There are many factors that either increase or decrease our risk of osteoporosis. Balanced nutrition along with a healthy and positive lifestyle are very effective strategies to prevent this and other health problems.

Breaking paradigms

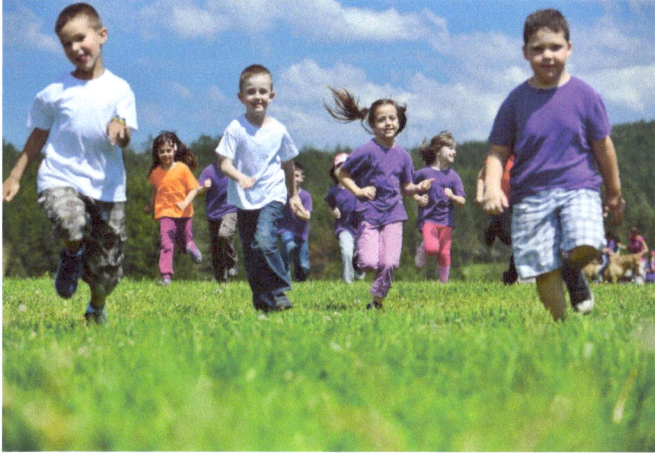

The whole issue around milk consumption leads me to think about the way we have been raised, with a series of mental conditionings that were instilled from an early age. Paradigms that we never thought to question or reconsider. Some of them come from our parents, grandparents and previous generations. But the world is changing, and what worked before may not apply to us anymore, because of the kind of life we lead, and the difference in the quality of the food we have available.

Other mental conditionings are triggered by society. Media advertising, the education given to us in school, and the influence we receive from our surroundings affect us directly. With advances in technology and communications, these have gained more and more power... we are constantly over-stimulated with information, images and concepts that end up being decisive in our view of life.

This constant stream of information is accompanied by an inevitable manipulation. For our family, it is an unconscious manipulation that affects us emotionally. In the second case, is has a strong component of commercial purposes.

Regardless of what lies behind all of these influences, the point is that they inevitably shape the way we think and act. I invite you to have an open mind, to learn, and also to unlearn, especially when it comes to your health. When we make a conscious effort to doubt and reevaluate those conditioning that we bring from the past as well as the information presented to us everyday, we can develop a clearer position about ourselves, and the world around us. This will translate in better decisions making for a healthier lifestyle.

In terms of nutrition, there may be as many diets, as people in the world, and it is up to each of us to determine, the type that will benefit us best.

Do not leave this important decision in the hands of others. Even though they may have the best intentions, our loved ones may have misconceptions or outdated ideas. Reevaluating those misconceptions can help not only us, but them as well. As far as the media goes, please keep in mind it is our food that is in question. It is best to question their campaigns and interests so that they won't tarnish our efforts to live a healthier lifestyle. We have the power and the right, to take responsibility for our own health.

No milk please

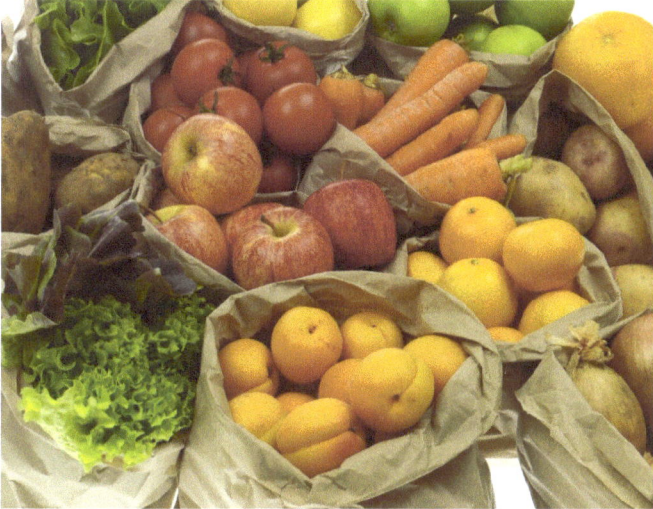

Returning to the starting point. More and more people are looking to reduce milk consumption while maintaining a healthy and balanced diet for a long and fulfilling life.

Remember that we are what we eat, and so, it is important to learn more about the relationship between our food and our health. Research different sources of advice, and select the information you want to embrace as part of your life.

By studying more on this topic, by learning to listen to your own body, and by discussing things with your health care professional or other experts in the field, you will be able to determine your specific nutritional needs. This will allow you to make better decisions about your diet and provide your body a healthier way of fueling itself. Start increasing consumption of natural foods and find the balance to feel good. How do you feel after eating a certain food? Being aware of this allows you to choose those things your body accepts better. And above all, make of this and any other changes in your life, an enjoyable process. Do not approach it as a punishment or a chore, but rather as a prize. You are deciding to give your body a better diet, because it deserves to be healthy and enjoy full energy and strength.

Specifically talking about milk and its substitutes, there are many vegetable milks to choose from. Embrace that spice that variety puts in life. My recommendation is to experience the different options until you find the ones you like the most, and best meet your dietary needs. Try consuming them in different ways; by themselves, or even combining some of them. Try them with cereal, in smoothies, or coffee. Many of them also work great in desserts and recipes that normally would have used cow's milk. Once vegetable milks become a part of your life, play with them in the kitchen coming up with new ideas; make them yourself at home, which adds that valuable ingredient of love and intention of health.

Vegetable Milks

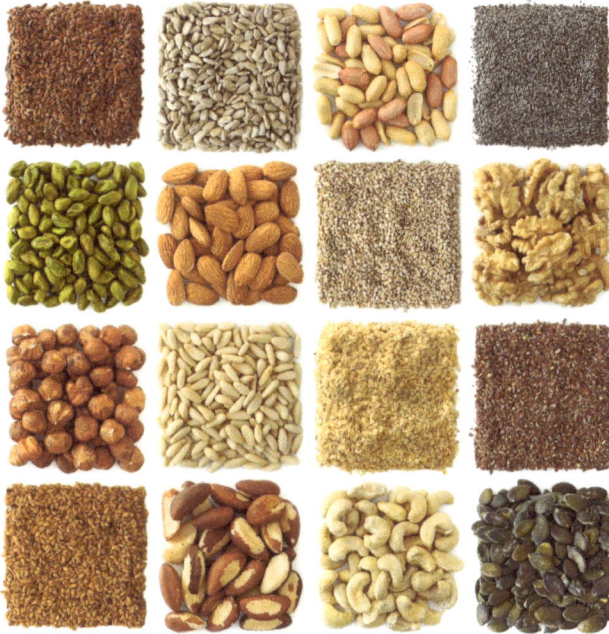

The strict meaning of the word "milk", refers only to that produced by mammals. However, this name has been used for certain vegetable beverages, because their appearance resemble said animal product. Call them milk, juices or extracts - these drinks are an excellent alternative to animal milks, both in taste and uses, and in nutritional value. For the purposes of this book, we will call them vegetable milks.

Vegetable milks can be made of grains, legumes, nuts and seeds... the possibilities are enormous. These drinks are delicious and have a number of health benefits such as providing excellent nutritional content - and at the same time, helping control fat and cholesterol levels and maintaining the body's mineral reserves. Vegetable milks, unlike the animal ones, have an alkalizing effect in the body. As we mentioned before, this means that they promote balance in our system, resulting in cell regeneration and disease prevention, slowing the aging process and increase the energy level.

Another advantage is that the vegetable milks are economical and can be prepared at home without specialized equipment. They are obtained from mixing the seed, grain or nut selected and water. Perhaps this is the shortest recipe, and the easiest to prepare recipe, that you can find in a book.

Using grains, milk can be made from barley or oats, among others. These are tasty and easy to prepare. Among legume milks, the most popular is soy, which we will discuss in more detail in the next chapter. My favorites are the milks of nuts or seeds. Among the first, are those of almonds, hazelnuts and cashews, to name a few. And among the seed, are hemp, quinoa, sesame and sunflower. Of course, each of these has a different nutritional value, depending on the product used as base. But since it has no additional ingredients or complicated processes, determining its nutritional value is actually quite easy: simply check the list of nutrients that the base product contains.

Soy milk

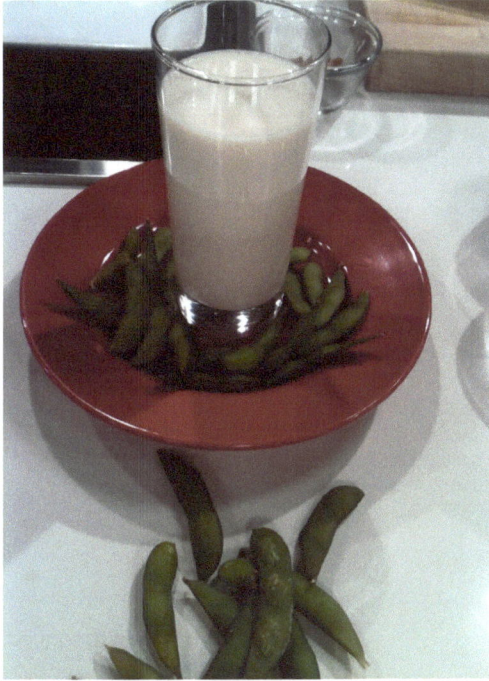

I would like to discuss soy milk first since it is the better known of all vegetable milks. It also happens to be the most controversial in terms of its effect on our health.

Soy milk has been widely used and marketed as the main alternative to animal milk. But it is far from an ideal alternative to dairy consumption. Not only because its taste is different and most people find it difficult to accept, but mostly because it may pose a threat of causing harmful effects to our health. The soy milk consumption has been associated with digestive problems like gas and stomach pains, disorders in addition to thyroid function and our reproductive system, especially in men.[6,61,62] It is important to note that of all grains, soybeans are the hardest to digest, and one of the more likely to produce intolerance or allergic processes when consumed.

Because of its high estrogen content, it has also been associated with an increased incidence of breast cancer, although there are opposing views on this matter.

One of the main reasons why soy milk is criticized, and many health experts prefer to stay away from it, is the controversy about genetically modified organisms. An estimated 90% of soybeans produced in the United States has been exposed to genetic manipulation.[6,75] Crops that have been treated in this way are sprayed with products designed to kill everything except the crop itself. Common sense necessarily suggests that what happens once these products enter our bodies is far from ideal.

For the reasons mentioned above, soy milk is not among my list of recommendations as a healthy alternative to dairy consumption. However, I do not want to generalize, because there are cases where control of GM crops is rather strict, eliminating that concern from the equation. Under this premise, even when there are concerns about its estrogen content, if it is consumed in moderation, it can be an interesting source of protein for some.

How to prepare vegetable milks

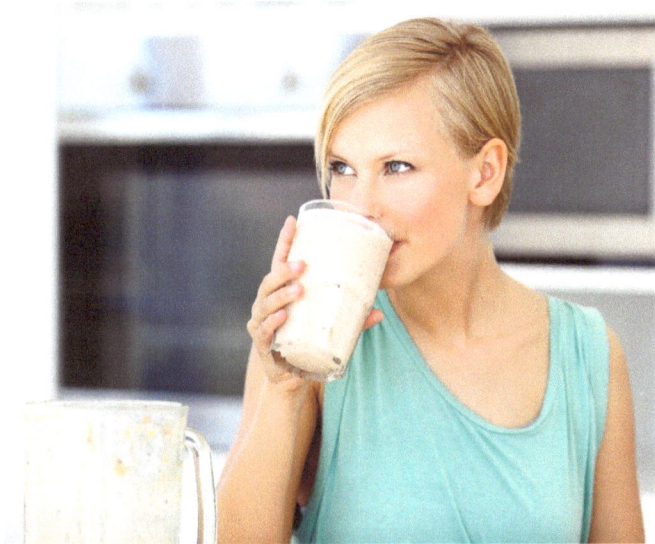

It is important to start off with nuts, grains and seeds in their natural state, not roasted or salted.

In the case of nuts and most seeds, the process is fairly simple. They should be soaked in water, preferably filtered after 8 to 12 hours (overnight, for example), depending on the milk you are preparing. The above is done with the purpose of softening the base product in order to facilitate blending, and ensuring that their nutrients are more bioavailable, or easy to absorb by the body. Once your base ingredient has softened, wash it and put it in the blender with filtered water. For each measure of nut or seed use between 2 and 3 parts water, depending on whether you want your beverage creamier or more liquid. Once blended, pass it through a very fine strainer or sieve. The pulp left in the strainer, can be blended again with a little more water, or stored in the refrigerator for later use in other recipes.

Milks of oats, barley or other grains are prepared similarly, without the need of soaking the grains for so long. Half an hour of soaking is enough. The oatmeal is one of the favorites in the group, for its extraordinary nutritional content, for its health benefits, and also for being fairly inexpensive and easy to find.

In the case of hemp, even though it is a seed, it does not require soaking, as it is quite soft. Easy to prepare and with unmatched nutritional value, hemp seed milk definitely has its place among my favorites.

Coconut milk does not require soaking either. It has a delicious taste, and offers great versatility when used as an ingredient in recipes, as do rice and nut milks. It is prepared by using coconut pulp and water. Part of the water can be replace with coconut water - rich in electrolytes and minerals.

Soy and other legume milks are slightly more elaborate; as it is recommended to remove the cuticles after soaking - since they can be heavy hard to digest - and to cook them, letting them boil for a few minutes, either before or after blending and straining. Cooking time varies depending on the type used and the preferences of the person who prepares it.

In any of the above cases, if desired, you can add a bit of agave or honey to sweeten and / or a pinch of Celtic salt for flavor. You may also add a few drops of vanilla or a little cinnamon. Some people like blending dates in them – a food with excellent nutritional content - or even lavender leaves to give it a more exotic flavor. This depends on your preferences. As you start preparing them, and playing with the flavor, you will develop your own recipes.

Since we have prepared milks that are 100% natural and free of preservatives, it is ideal to consume them fresh. But if you would rather make more, they can also be refrigerated and kept for a maximum of 2 to 3 days.

Hydration, hydration, hydration

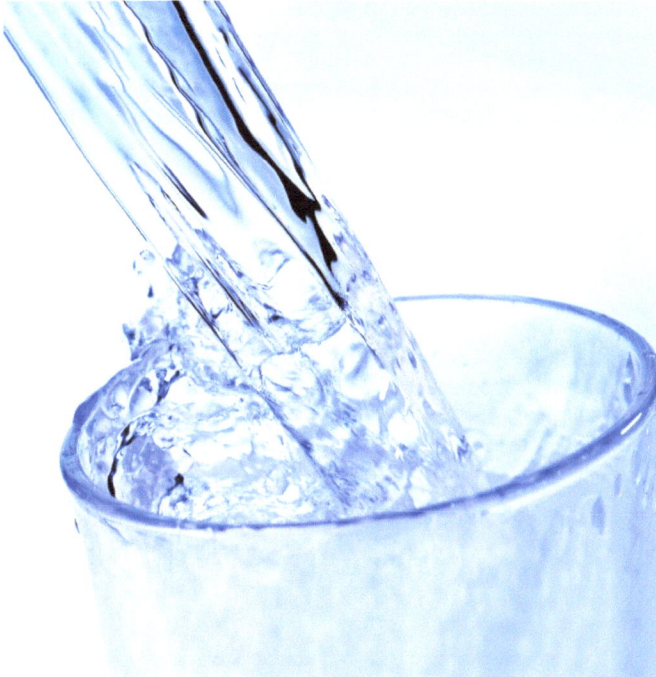

One cannot speak of milk or any nutritional practice without discussing the issue of hydration. The reason being, it determines to a large extent our overall health.

We have referred to the importance of maintaining enough oxygen circulating in the body, to maintain a balance and protect our health. This concept is directly linked with the importance of staying hydrated. A high percentage of us live dehydrated, which is the cause of many of our health conditions. But opposite to popular belief, it is not a matter of just drinking plenty of fluids, since not everyone hydrate our body. In fact, the vast majority has the opposite effect at the cellular level.

When we drink coffee, alcohol, carbonated beverages, sports or sugary drinks, and even cow's milk, we are in some way dehydrating our body. So when you think about hydration, instead of going for one of these drinks, look for a glass of water. Water, specifically that with a higher pH (also known as alkaline), is the best way to hydrate the body.[63] It is not a bad idea, when we do consume any of the drinks mentioned before, to accompany it with a glass of pure water. Without going into technical details, the problem with the drinks listed above, is that when consumed, the body needs to convert their sugars into glucose in order to transport them through our system. This depletes water from the body's reserves. These drinks act as diuretics; draining water from our system. In that case, ironically, the beverages we drink, are highly responsible for our dehydration.

Dehydration has been associated with many current diseases.[64,65] Even though water is not the focus of this book, it is so important that I could not leave it out of these lines. Many people struggle to lose weight, to prevent the constant colds and respiratory illnesses, to care for their skin, hair and nails. And we do not realize that one of the best tools to achieve those goals is very much at hand. Make water your best ally in health. And if you don't have the habit of consuming it, I suggest you start working on it. The idea is not to drink 8 glasses of water in one sitting. Rather, do it all along your day and you will be drinking more and more water without really noticing. When we have a glass of water on the desk, or at hand during the day and take a little here and a little there, it slowly starts to turn into a routine, and without realizing, we significantly increased our level of hydration.

One of the reasons why many of us live chronically dehydrated is because our body shows no sign of this condition until it has reached a fairly advanced level. When we feel thirsty or have a dry mouth, our organism has reached a high degree of dehydration. What I mean by this is that we were dehydrated long before those signs started to show. There are other, less evident, signs our body sends us, but most people do not associate them with dehydration. Such signs are fatigue, lack of energy and light sleep, among others.

Did you know that dehydration could cause cravings?[6] Many times, our body is dehydrated, but instead of sending us the message of it being thirsty, it transmits it as a whim. Sweet cravings or wanting more salt in our meals are considered by some experts as signs of dehydration. So the next time this happens, drink a glass of water and give your body a few minutes to determine how real was this "caprice".

The minimum recommendation is to drink the equivalent to half of your weight (in pounds) in ounces of water. That is if you weigh for example 160 pounds, the ideal is to drink at least 80 ounces of water. If you calculate your weight in kilos, then the number on the scale should be the minimum number of ounces of water you drink daily. Note that I have mentioned that this recommendation amounts to a basic consumption. Ideally, your water intake should be greater than that estimate, especially if you live in warmer climates, or if your levels of physical activity or stress are high.

A good way to spice up the water and at the same time increase its alkalizing benefits is by adding a few drops of lemon or lime to it. These two specific fruits have excellent qualities, both in terms of balance in pH and detoxifying properties. A glass of water with lemon in the morning, warm or at room temperature can be a great ally when looking to lose weight, or rid the body of toxins when we have had days of poor diet or high anxiety.

Although it is recommended to drink water throughout the day, perhaps the most important glass of water everyday is right when you wake up in the morning. Our body naturally wakes up dehydrated after sleeping for several hours. Similarly, one should consume more water when we sweat or lose body fluids, when we spent some time in the sun, doing physical work or exercising.

Conclusion

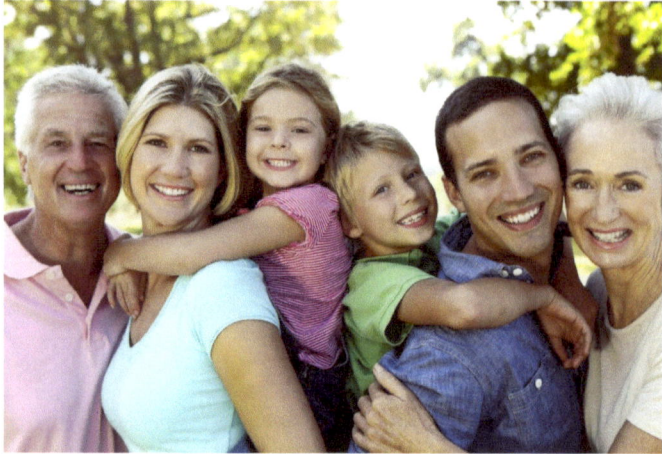

Everyone is the owner and author of his/her own health. And while it is impossible to control 100% of what happens in our body, it is feasible to increase the chances of a long and healthy life, and reduce the risk of disease and decay through good nutrition and a healthy lifestyle.

It is worth keeping in mind that our body functions in a very basic manner. It is made to understand and assimilate certain types of nutrition, and faces great challenges when fed with food and drink that it does not recognize as part of its natural diet.

As mentioned, the pace of development of the food industry has radically influenced our habits, and our body has failed to keep up. Evolutionary processes are slow and when we do not allow the body to take time to adjust to new conditions, we begin to see the consequences in the form of disease and dysfunction.

We live in a society with a very difficult health situation. Diabetes, cancer and heart disease's statistics have exploded and now affect a high percentage of our population. That is why today, more than ever, it is crucial to take our health into our own hands and become conscious about good nutrition, with an open mind to learn and unlearn, to auto-evaluate ourselves and to find those things in our routine, we could change or improve.

I wish you HEALTH, HAPPINESS and JOY today and always. And I hope your appetite to learn grows every day. Information is power!

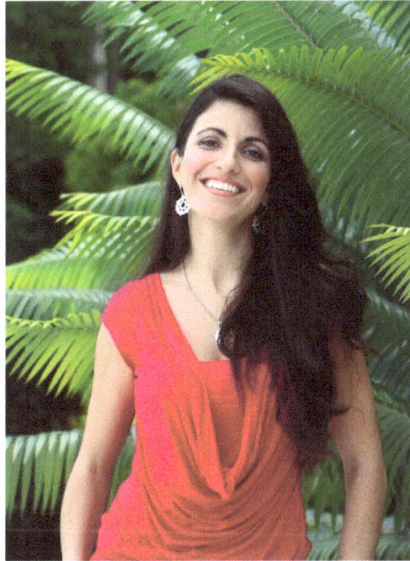

Recipes

Almond milk rice pudding

- Courtesy of Paula Smith-Labbad

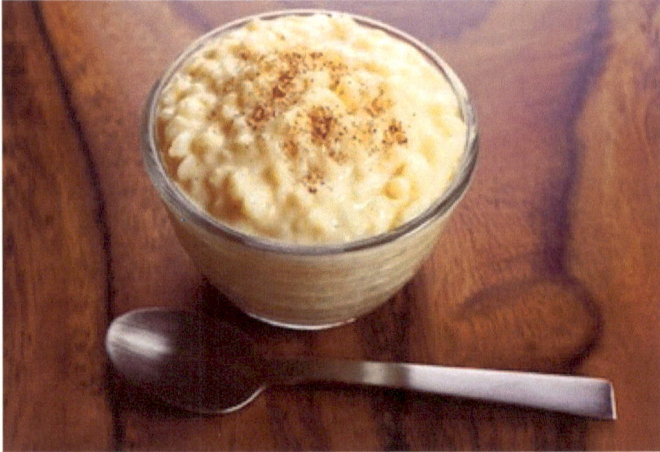

Portions - 6

This is a delicious way to vary the recipe of the traditional rice pudding to make it dairy free.

Ingredients:

1 Cup Valence rice	
1 Cup agave	
1 Liter Almond Milk	
3 Cinnamon sticks	

Preparation:

Mix the ingredients and cook over medium heat for 30 minutes. Allow cooling, and then refrigerating covered. You can decorate with cinnamon powder before serving.

Variation:

This recipe can also be prepared using sugar instead of agave, but I recommend the latter, for its taste and especially because it is a much healthier alternative to refined sugar.

Chia Seed Pudding with Hemp Seed

- Courtesy of Chef Elena Dal Forno
www.Facebook.com/RawVeganChefElena

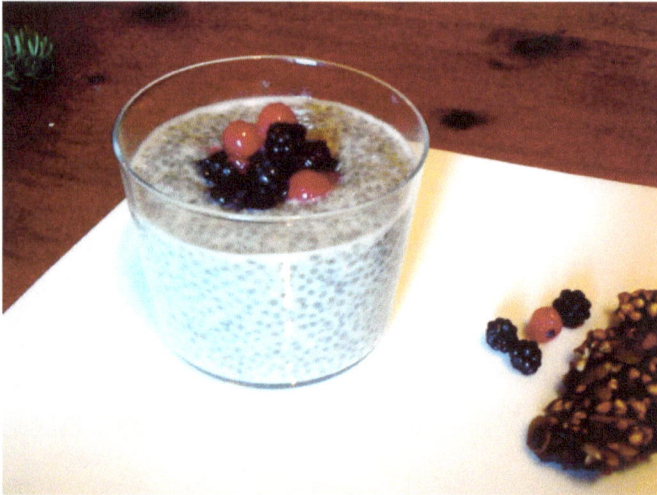

Before going to the recipe, I want to give a well-deserved introduction to the protagonist of the same. Chia seed (Salvia hispanica) has been used by the Aztecs as a source of energy and nutrition from pre-Columbian times. It has great content of minerals, amino acids and omega 3 besides being one of the best sources of gelatinous fiber. This makes it not only a great food, but also a great alternative to cleanse and detoxify the body, while helping improve the functioning of the digestive system.

Portions – 2

Chef Elena comments: "Although this is a recipe that works well with almost any kind of nut milk, I must admit that my favorite milks for this one are pistachio, almond, coconut and hemp seeds. So in this case I used hemp seeds that give milk a rich, creamy flavor, plus you don't even have to strain it! Also, because hemp is full with omegas so you get all the good stuff!"

Milk preparation:

Ingredients:

2 Cups of filtered water
1/3 to 1/2 Cup of hemp seed (depending on how "rich" you want it.

Blend in a high-speed blender until the seeds are completely crushed.

To assemble:

Ingredients:

2 Cups of hemp seed
1 Banana
2 TBSP agave (or the sweetener of your choice)
1/2 TBSP Vanilla
A pinch of salt
1/2 Cup of chia seeds

Blend together all the ingredients except for the chia seeds. Once you are done pour the liquid into a bowl and pour the chia seeds over it. Cover with a cling film and let it sit in the fridge for an hour. Chia seeds will quadruple their size in that time and firm up the mix. Serve with some banana slices or mixed berries on top, and some granola if you have it. This is for me the perfect breakfast!

Iced Mate Latte

- Courtesy of Chef Barry Kraemer <ins>www.ChefKraemer.com</ins>

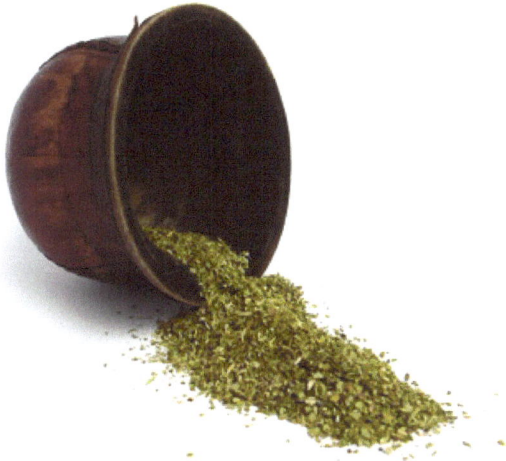

Portions: 2

Ingredients:

5 + 1/2 TBSP of Yerba Mate
2 Cups of water
1 + 3/4 Cups of coconut milk
1 Cup of ice
4 TBSP dark agave nectar
3/4 TBSP ground cinnamon
1 TBSP ground cardamom

2 pinches salt

Brew 5 +1/2 Tbsp. Yerba Mate in French Press for 7 minutes, allow to cool.

Once it is cold, mix with the rest of the ingredients. Blend in large blender, and enjoy.

"The Natural"

Courtesy of Chef David Choi

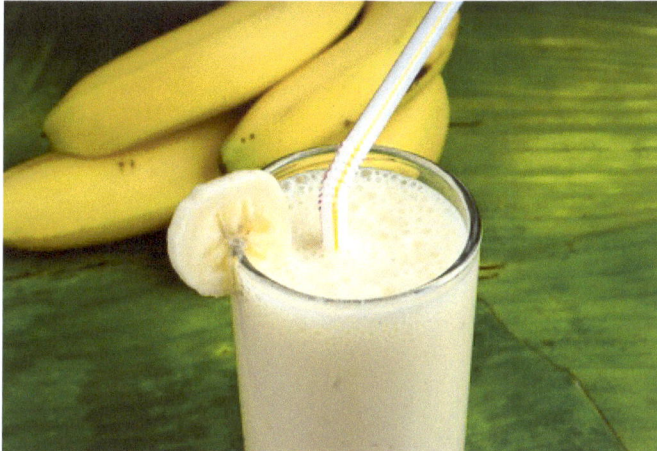

Chef David recommends using organic ingredients.

Portions: 1

Ingredients:

1 1/2 cups of unsweetened almond, rice or soy milk
1 Banana
1/5 of brick of tofu
1/2 Avocado
1/2 Cup of mango / papaya / peaches / persimmon
1/2 Cup blueberries or strawberries

1/4 Cup of walnuts or 1-2 TBS pine nuts

Blend all ingredients in a blender and enjoy right away. Adjust thickness by adding more or less non-dairy milk. This drink is packed with antioxidants, vitamins, minerals, and protein. Enjoy!

Renowned professional athletes around the world have used this recipe as a natural energy drink.

Cold Cauliflower-Coconut Soup

Courtesy of Mel, with Balance pH-Diet – <u>www.Balance-pH-Diet.com</u>

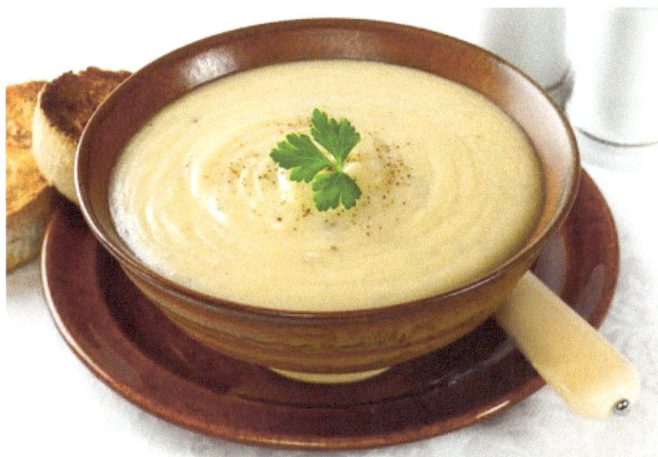

Mel mentions in her recipe: "Besides being an alkaline food, cauliflowers also have several other health benefits including: improving heart health, reducing the risk of strokes and strengthen the immune system. Cauliflower can also help to prevent colon cancer and maintain healthy cholesterol levels. Fresh coconut milk is full of Lauric Acids, which makes it anti-carcinogenic, anti-microbial, anti-bacterial as well as anti-viral. Coconut milk can help to fight off all sorts of viruses and help to lower cholesterol as well as to prevent cancer."

Portions: 4

Ingredients:

1 Pound fresh cauliflower
1 + 1/4 Cup unsweetened coconut

milk	
1 Cup of water	
2 TBSP fresh lime juice	
1/3 Cup cold pressed extra virgin olive oil	
1/2 Cup fresh coriander leaves, chopped	
Pinch of salt and cayenne pepper	
1 handful of unsweetened coconut chips	

Directions:

Steam cauliflower for around 10 minutes.

Then, put the cauliflower together with coconut milk and water in a food processor and process until very smooth. Add fresh lime juice, salt and pepper, most of the chopped coriander and the oil and mix for another few seconds.

Pour in soup bowls and garnish with coriander and coconut chips. Enjoy!

Oven-Roasted Vegetables with Thai Coconut Curry Sauce

Courtesy of Chef Erik Mathes, http://www.linkedin.com/in/erikmathes

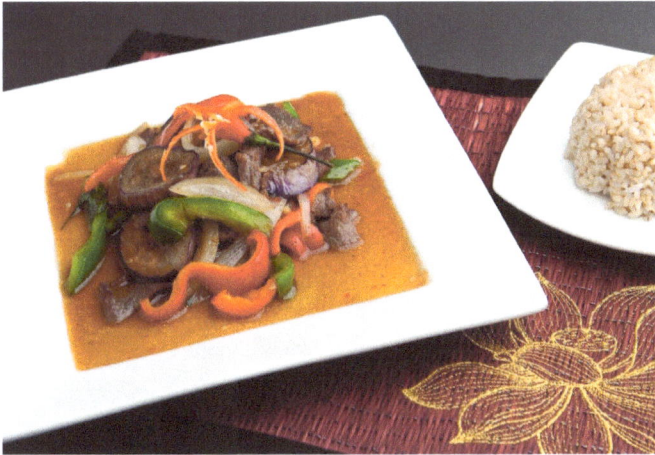

Portions: 8 a 10

Ingredients:

1 head of cauliflower, cut into florets
1 head of broccoli, cut into florets
1 sweet onion, cut into large chunks
2 red bell peppers, cut into large squares
1 small bag of baby carrots
3 to 4 TBSP avocado, canola, or other neutral oil
1 TBSP ground cumin

1 TBSP ground coriander
1 TBSP granulated garlic
1 TBSP generic curry powder, garam masala, or your favorite curry blend
2 TBSP light or dark brown sugar
Kosher salt and cracked black pepper, to taste

Coconut curry sauce:

1 TBSP avocado, canola or neutral oil
1 shallot, finely chopped
2 cloves of garlic, finely chopped
3 cans of coconut milk (please do not use reduced fat coconut milk!)
2 TBSP Thai red curry paste
1 TBSP fish sauce (optional); substitute with salt, soy sauce, or liquid aminos
3 TBSP sugar (granulated or turbinado; traditional Thai cuisine calls for palm sugar -- use this if you can find it/prefer it)
2 TBSP roasted red chili paste (Thai Kitchen brand; optional)
Kosher salt and cracked black pepper, to taste (optional)
Fresh lime juice, to taste

Procedure:

Pre-heat oven to 425 ºF. Cut vegetables and measure ingredients to recipe specs. In a large mixing bowl, toss cut vegetables with oil and spice mixture until evenly coated. Use more oil if necessary, and try to break up sugar clumps as best as possible.

Arrange vegetables on foil-lined baking sheet or in roasting pan and cook until slightly charred and caramelized, about 20 minutes. You want a little bit of blackened, especially the edges of the broccoli florets -- delicious!

Meanwhile, while the vegetables roast, start the sauce:

Place your saucepot on the stove over medium heat; add the oil and then cook the shallot and garlic for 1 to 2 minutes, taking care not to burn them. Add the coconut milk and bring up to a boil; turn temperature down to a simmer once it starts boiling to avoid any boiling over.

In a small bowl, add the red curry paste and pour a ladle or so full of the hot coconut milk over it. Mix them together with a fork until curry paste is uniformly blended into milk and then add it back into the rest of the coconut milk mixture. Add the fish sauce or substitute, sugar, and roasted red chili paste and continue to cook over medium-low to medium heat, whisking occasionally until the sauce thickens up.

Once the sauce is thick enough to coat the back of a spoon, taste it and add salt and black pepper to your taste, and then add a few squirts of fresh lime juice to your liking.

Ideally, the vegetables and sauce will be ready at the same time. Carefully take the veggies out of the oven, and serve them with a coating of the coconut curry sauce and a side of jasmine or basmati rice.

Smoothie with a wine surprise

- Courtesy of Chef Elena Dal Forno
www.Facebook.com/RawVeganChefElena

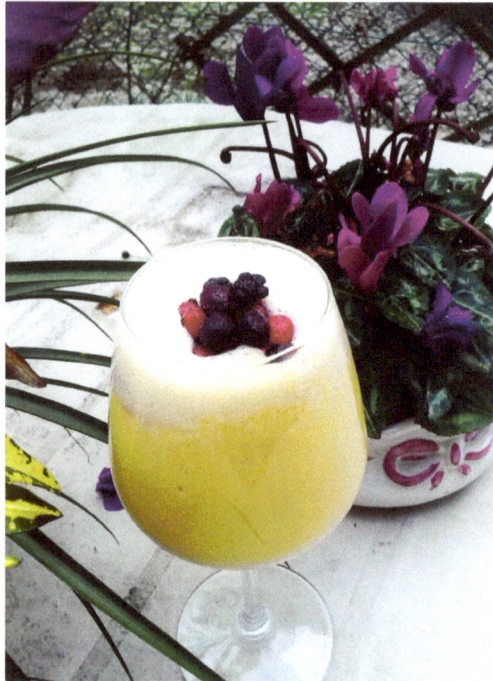

Portions: 1

Ingredients:

1 + 1/2 Almond milk
1 Mango roughly chopped
1/4 Cup pineapple

1 TBSP lemon juice
1 Tsp maple syrup (optional)
1/2 Tsp vanilla extract
1/2 Cup of frozen wild berries (blueberry and blackberry are perfect)
A pinch of salt
Some sprigs of fresh rosemary to garnish (optional)

Directions:

Blend the mango and 1 cup of almond milk and pour the liquid into a big wine glass. Then blend the pineapple with a 1/4 cup of milk and pour on top to create a "second" layer.

Then blend really well 1/4 cup of frozen berries and 1/4 cup of the milk left and pour the black liquid in the middle of your smoothie, to create a "wine" surprise in the middle. Garnish the top with other berries and enjoy!

Almond milk flan

Courtesy of Marie Baccini

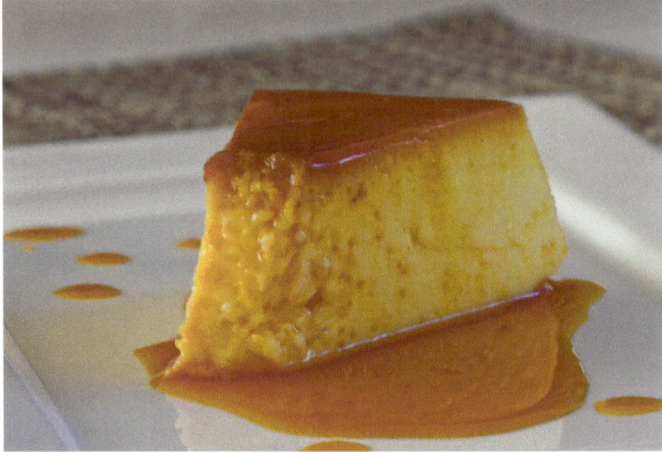

Portions: 8

Ingredients:

2 Cups almond milk
4 Eggs
4 Egg yolks
1/2 Cup of sugar
1 Can of coconut milk
Optional: orange or lemon zest and / or vanilla extract
Drops of lemon

Directions for the Flan:

First prepare the caramel: Place the sugar with a few drops of lemon juice in a saucepan over medium heat until it reaches caramel consistency. Do not let it get too dark as it becomes bitter. Pour the caramel onto the bottom of the pan or mold that will be used.

Blend milk, eggs, egg yolks and orange or lemon zest and / or vanilla extract. Pour on top of the caramel into the pan and bake-bath. This cooking method involves placing the vessel into a larger vessel with water, and place both in the oven. Bake at 375 ºF for half an hour. Let cool to room temperature before refrigerating.

Serve with coconut milk whipped cream.

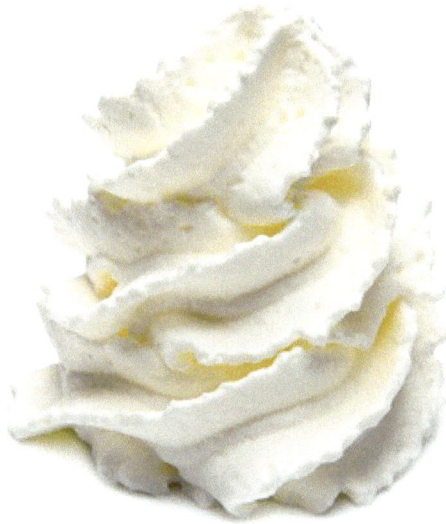

Directions for the coconut milk whipped cream:

Refrigerate a can of coconut milk for 24 hours. At the time of use, flip the can so you open the bottom end of it. The milk will be separated into a thick part and a liquid part. Use only the thick and beat with a hand mixer until you have the desired consistency, and can use it to decorate the dessert.

Alkaline Pumpkin Coconut Soup

Courtesy of Mel, with Balance pH Diet - www.Balance-pH-Diet.com

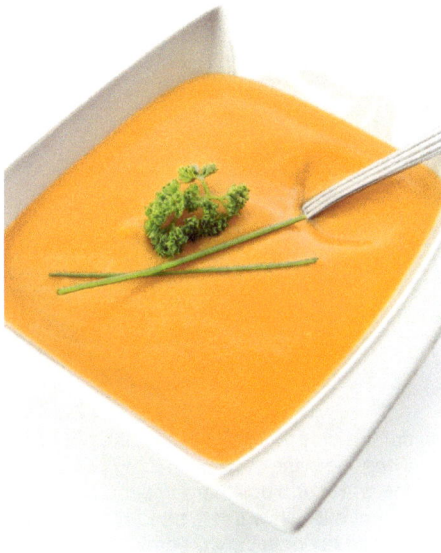

Mel reminds us: Pumpkins are not only alkaline, but also very low in calories, which make them an ideal vegetable for anybody who watches its weight. Moreover, pumpkins are rich in potassium, magnesium, zinc, fiber, iron as well as beta-carotene (antioxidant), which are really good at neutralizing free radicals."

Portions: 4

Ingredients

2 lb pumpkin
6 Cups of water
1 Cup of coconut milk
5 ounces potatoes
2 big onions
3 ounces leek
1 handful of fresh parsley
1 pinch of nutmeg
1 pinc of cayenne pepper
1 Tsp sea salt
4 TBSP cold pressed extra virgin olive oil

Directions:

First of all: cut the onions, the pumpkin, the potatoes as well as the leek into small pieces. Then, heat the olive oil in a big pot and sauté the onions for a few minutes. Add the water and boil the pumpkin, potatoes and the leek until tender. Add the coconut milk. Now use a hand blender and puree for around 1 minute. The soup should become very creamy.

Season with salt, pepper and nutmeg and finally add the Parsley. Enjoy this alkalizing pumpkin soup hot or cold!

Vegan Coconut Flan

- Courtesy of Chef Barry Kraemer www.ChefKraemer.com

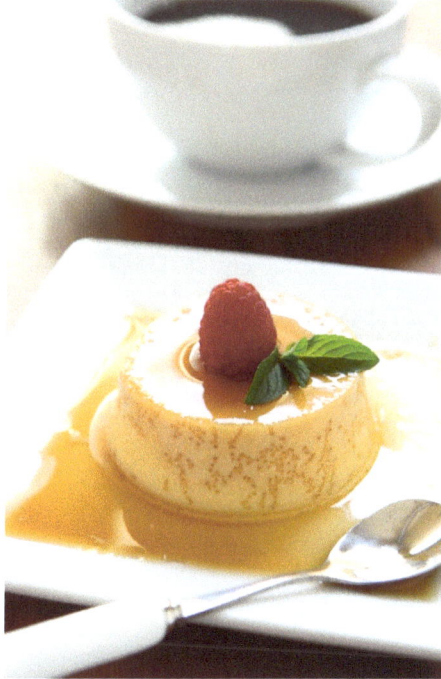

Portions: 8

1/2 Cup Natural Sugar (Demerra or Turbinado is best)
2 TBSP rum
4 TBSP Agar-Agar (Vegan gelatin from seaweed)
3 Cans of coconut milk
1/2 Tsp Sea salt

1/4 Tsp Turmeric
12 oz. Silken Tofu
2/3 Cups sugar
2 TBSP + 1 Tsp Vanilla extract
2 TBSP Corn, potato or tapioca starch

Directions:

In a small stainless steel or nonstick skillet, heat the sugar on medium-low heat—you don't want to burn the sugar, but caramelize it. Do not stir with a spoon; don't do anything except watch it. This should take about five minutes. As it starts to brown and form syrup, add the rum and cook until the mixture is thick and syrupy. Pour immediately into a round shallow cake pan, or glass-baking dish, like a soufflé dish or a pie plate, and swirl it around to evenly coat the bottom. Preheat the oven to 350 ºF.

Meanwhile in a small sauce pan add 1 cup of the coconut milk with the agar-agar and heat to a low boil, then turn the heat to low, add in the salt and turmeric and whisk, then simmer for five minutes.

In a blender, add the tofu, sugar and 2 cups of the coconut milk and blend until incorporated. Heat the cornstarch with the remaining coconut milk in a small saucepan on medium heat until it reaches a slow boil, stirring often.

Add to the blender the heated agar and cornstarch mixtures and blend until well incorporated. This is your custard.

Pour the custard over the sugar in the pan. Place the baking dish inside of a large roasting pan and set in the oven. Fill the outer pan with boiling water to 1 inch deep.

Bake for 25 minutes, this melts the caramel into the custard a bit. You don't need to bake it as long as a typical custard because there are no eggs, so remove the pan and let it cool for 45 minutes, then let it cool in the refrigerator for at least two hours to set, better overnight.

Run a butter knife around the edges of the baking dish to loosen the flan, then turn over onto a serving dish, and then cut into slices and serve. You can also bake these in individual large ceramic ramekins.

Serve with chopped pineapple, strawberries, blackberries or other fresh fruit.

Red beet and radicchio soup

- Courtesy of Chef Elena Dal Forno
<u>**www.Facebook.com/RawVeganChefElena**</u>

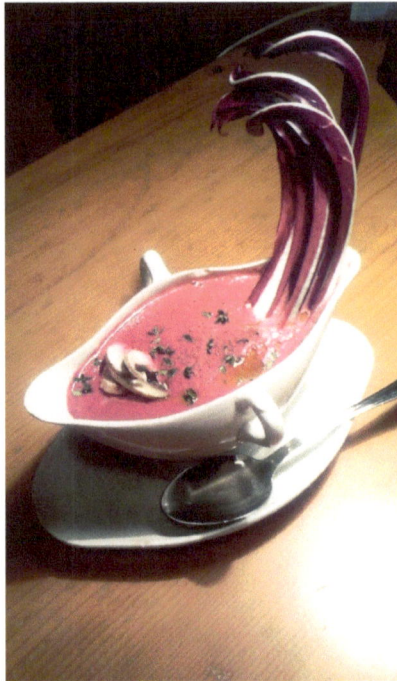

Chef Elena considers this one of her favorite soup in the winter, for its extraordinary color and nutritional content. If you do not have radicchio, soup can be prepared without it.

This soup really works well with coconut milk but also almond milk, walnut milk or Brazilian nut milk work very well.

Ingredients:

2 + 1/2 Cups coconut milk.
1 Red beet, not too big
1/2 Cup of radicchio
1/2 Cup raw cashews, more if you want it thicker, or substitute with 1 avocado
1/4 Cup red onion or 1 Tsp onion powder
2-3 TBSP extra virgin olive oil
1 clove garlic (optional)
1 Tsp curry (optional)
Salt and pepper to taste

Blend everything to reach a creamy consistence. Garnish with some fresh thyme or oregano, some radicchio leaves and some mushrooms previously marinated in tamari and olive oil. If you want you can even warm it up a little bit... Enjoy!

References

1. Ferguson, James D., VMD, MS. "Milk Protein." *Penn Veterinary Medicine, Center for Animal Health and Productivity.* N.p., n.d. Web. <http://research.vet.upenn.edu/DairyPoultrySwine/DairyCattle/MUN/MilkProtein/tabid/1595/Default.aspx>.

2. Schmidt, Erica. "Aspectos Ambientales Vinculados Con La Industria Láctea."*Instituto Nacional De Tecnología Industrial.* Ministerio De Industria Y Turismo, Secretaria de Industria, Comercio y de La Pequeña y Mediana Empresa, n.d. Web. <http://www.inti.gov.ar/lacteos/pdf/aspectos.pdf>.

3. Lobo Poblet, María S. "Informe Aspectos Ambientales, Sociales Y Económicos Industria Láctea." *Ministerio De Industria.* Secretaría De Industria, Jan. 2009. Web. <http://www.sic.gob.ar/uma/wp-content/uploads/2010/01/informe-industria-lactea.pdf>.

4. Powers, Wendy. "Environmental Challenges Ahead for the U.S. Dairy Industry." *Florida Dairy Extension.* University of Florida, 28 Apr. 2009. Web. 09 Dec. 2012. <http://dairy.ifas.ufl.edu/dpc/2009/Powers.pdf>.

5. Capper, J. L., R.A., and Cady and D. E. Bauman. "The Environmental Impact of Dairy Production: 1944 Compared with 2007." *Journal of Animal Science* (2009): n. pag. *Advantages of Domestic Species and Dual -Purpose Models That Benefit Agricultural and Biomedical Research.* J Anim Sci, 13 Mar. 2009. Web. <http://www.adsbm.msu.edu/Portals/0/2009%20Capper%20et%20al_1944%20vs%202007%20Carbon%20Footprintas%202009-1781v1.pdf>.

6. Rosenthal, Joshua. *Integrative Nutrition: Feed Your Hunger for Health and Happiness.* New York, NY: Integrative Nutrition Pub., 2008. Print.

7. Lear, Jessica. "Our Furry Friends, the History of Animal Domestication." *Journal of Young Investigators* 23.1 (n.d.): n. pag. *Journal of Young Investigators.* Journal of Young Investigators, Mar. 2012. Web. <http://www.jyi.org/news/nb.php?id=3769>.

8. "Historical Timeline - Milk - ProCon.org." *Historical Timeline - Milk - ProCon.org.* ProCon.org, 25 Aug. 2011. Web. <http://milk.procon.org/view.resource.php?resourceID=000832>.

9. Cellania, Miss. "Neatorama." *Neatorama.* N.p., 31 Mar. 2011. Web. <http://www.neatorama.com/2011/03/31/the-history-of-dairy-products/>.

10. Campbell, Dr. T Colin. "T. Colin Campbell Foundation." *T. Colin Campbell Foundation.* N.p., 2008. Web. <http://www.tcolincampbell.org/>.

11. "Health Concerns about Dairy Products." *PCRM*. Physicians Committee of Responsible Medicine, n.d. Web. <http://pcrm.org/search/?cid=252>.

12. Campbell, T. Colin, and Thomas M. Campbell. The China Study: The Most Comprehensive Study of Nutrition Ever Conducted and the Startling Implications for Diet, Weight Loss and Long-term Health. Dallas, TX: BenBella, 2005. Print.

13. Group III, Dr. Edward F., DC, ND. "Pasteurized vs. Raw Milk: Which One Is Healthier for You & Your Family?" *Natural Health Organic Living Blog*. N.p., 28 Sept. 2009. Web. <http://www.globalhealingcenter.com/natural-health/raw-milk-vs-pasteurized-milk/>.

14. McAfee, Marl. "The 15 Things That Milk Pasteurization Kills." *The 15 Things That Pasteurization Kills*. N.p., 3 Aug. 2010. Web. <http://www.realmilk.com/15-things-milk-pasteurization-kills.html>.

15. Sarria Ruiz, Beatriz. "Efectos Del Tratamiento Térmico De Fórmulas Infantiles Y Leche De Vaca Sobre La Biodisponibilidad Mineral Y Protéica." Thesis. Universidad Complutense, 1998. *E-Prints Complutense*. Biblioteca Universidad Complutense. Web. <http://eprints.ucm.es/tesis/19972000/X/3/X3068001.pdf>.

16. Enig, Aru G., PhD. "Milk Homogenization and Heart Disease." *Real Milk Articles*. N.p., 13 Dec. 2003. Web. <http://www.realmilk.com/homogenization.html>.

17. Grant, Irene R., Alan G. Williams, Michael T. Rowe, and D. Donald Muir. "Efficacy of Various Pasteurization Time-Temperature Conditions in Combination with Homogenization on Inactivation of Mycobacterium Avium Subsp. Paratuberculosis in Milk." *Applied and Environmental Microbiology* (2005): n. pag. *U.S. National Library of Medicine, National Institute of Health*. Web. <http://www.ncbi.nlm.nih.gov/pmc/articles/PMC1151836/>.

18. Cohen, Robert. "Homogenized Milk: Rocket Fuel for Cancer." *Health 101*. N.p., n.d. Web. <http://www.health101.org/art_milk_cancer_fuel.htm,>.

19. Whittekin, Martie, CCN. "Our Diet Has Changed More in the Last 100 Years than in the Previous 10,000!" *Radio Martie*. N.p., 2002. Web. <http://www.radiomartie.com/articles/history_of_food_chart.pdf>.

20. "How the Western Diet Has Changed in Nutrition and Calories." *Complete Health Improvement Program*. Lifestyle Medicine Institute, n.d. Web. <http://www.chiphealth.com/health_topics/topics/trends_in_dietary_changes.php>.

21. "Dairy Investigation | Mercy For Animals." *Mercy For Animals*. N.p., n.d. Web. <http://www.mercyforanimals.org/dairy/>.

22. "Dairy Production on Factory Farms." *Farm Sanctuary*. N.p., n.d. Web. <http://www.farmsanctuary.org/learn/factory-farming/dairy/,>.

23. Bedard, Megan. "5 Dirty Secrets of the Dairy Industry." *Take Part*. N.p., n.d. Web. <http://www.takepart.com/article/2012/04/12/5-things-you-dont-know-about-dairy-industry>.

24. "Overview of the United States Dairy Industry." *United States Department of Agriculture - Economics, Statistics and Market Information System*. USDA, 22 Sept. 2010. Web. <http://usda.mannlib.cornell.edu/usda/current/USDairyIndus/USDairyIndus-09-22-2010.pdf>.

25. Hoskin, Roger. "Farm Milk Production." *USDA Economic Research Service*. N.p., 22 June 2012. Web. <http://www.ers.usda.gov/topics/animal-products/dairy/background.aspx>.

26. "The Industrial Milk Factory; It's No Dairy." *Factory Farming*. N.p., n.d. Web. <http://www.factory-farming.com/milk_factory.html>.

27. "30 Razones Para No Ingerir Leche De Vaca | Mente Vegana." *Mente Vegana*. N.p., n.d. Web. <http://www.mentevegana.org/30-razones-para-no-ingerir-secrecion-mamaria-leche-de-vaca.html>.

28. "Veganismo En Conciencia De Krishna." *VEGAN PRASADAM*. N.p., 6 Sept. 2011. Web. <http://veganprasadam.blogspot.com/2011/09/ingredientes-2-tazas-200ml-de-agua-4.html>.

29. Harry. "Los Riesgos De Tomar Leche De Vaca." *Cuerpo Armonioso*. N.p., 17 Aug. 2010. Web. <http://www.cuerpoarmonioso.com/2010/08/los-riesgos-de-tomar-leche-de-vaca/>.

30. Elliott, Stuart. "ADVERTISING; When Doctors, and Even Santa, Endorsed Tobacco."*The New York Times*. The New York Times, 07 Oct. 2008. Web. <http://www.nytimes.com/2008/10/07/business/media/07adco.html>.

31. Jones, Dr. Daemon. "Milk or Green Leafy Vegetables: Which Is Better for Calcium Absorption?" *EnpowerHER*. N.p., 15 Nov. 2011. Web. <http://www.empowher.com/bones-amp-joints/content/milk-or-green-leafy-vegetables-which-better-calcium-absorption>.

32. Palafox, Jorge Carlos. "Las Mejores Fuentes De Calcio." Editorial. *Discovery DSalud*Mar. 2010: n. pag. *DISCOVERY DSALUD*. MK3 S.L.C. Web. <http://www.dsalud.com/index.php?pagina=articulo>.

33. Boyles, Salynn. "Study: Calcium May Increase Heart Attack Risk." *WebMD*. WebMD, 29 July 2010. Web.

<http://www.webmd.com/heart/news/20100729/study-calcium-may-increase-heart-attack-risk>.

34. "Dispatch: Have A Heart, Dont Eat Calcium Supplements." *ACSH*. N.p., 30 July 2010. Web. <http://www.acsh.org/factsfears/newsID.1703/news_detail.asp>.

35. Johnson, Megan. "Health Buzz: Calcium Supplements May Boost Heart Attack Risk."*US News*. U.S.News & World Report, 30 July 2010. Web. <http://health.usnews.com/health-news/family-health/heart/articles/2010/07/30/health-buzz-calcium-supplements-may-boost-heart-attack-risk>.

36. Freeman, Andrew, and Christina Kharbertyan. "18 'Food, Inc.' Facts Everyone Should Know." *News, Lifestyle, and Social Action on TakePart*. N.p., 24 Oct. 2012. Web. <http://www.takepart.com/photos/food-inc-facts/factory-farms-dominate>.

37. "Facts About the Poultry Industry." *Born Free USA*. N.p., n.d. Web. <http://www.bornfreeusa.org/facts.php?more=1&p=374>.

38. Sears, Dr. William. "Farmed Fish vs. Wild Fish." *Ask Dr. Sears*. N.p., n.d. Web. <http://www.askdrsears.com/topics/family-nutrition/fish/farmed-fish-vs-wild-fish>.

39. Emily, Main. "This or That: Wild vs. Farmed Fish." *Rodale*. N.p., n.d. Web. <http://www.rodale.com/wild-or-farmed-fish>.

40. Shor, Jamie. "First Global Study Reveals Health Risks OfWidely Eaten Farm Raised Salmon." *Institute for Health and the Environment*. University at Albany, n.d. Web. <http://www.albany.edu/ihe/salmonstudy/pressrelease.html>.

41. "Farm-raised or Wild Fish: What's the Difference?" *Eco Evaluator*. N.p., n.d. Web. <http://www.ecoevaluator.com/lifestyle/smart-food/farm-raised-or-wild-fish-whats-the-difference.html>.

42. "Hemp Benefits." *Living Harvest Tempt*. N.p., n.d. Web. <http://www.livingharvest.com/eating-hemp/benefits>.

43. Osburn, Lynn. "HEMP SEED: The Most Nutritionally Complete Food Source In The World." *Hemp Line Journal* 1.1 (1992): 14-15. *Ratical*. Web. <http://www.ratical.org/renewables/hempseed1.html>.

44. Leson, Gero. "Nutritional Profile and Benefits of Hemp Seed, Nut and Oil." *Dr. Bronner's Magic All-One*. N.p., n.d. Web. <http://www.drbronner.com/pdf/hempnutrition.pdf>.

45. Ponds, Amielia. "Hemp Protein: Eat the Nutrients." *Natural News*. N.p., 9 Dec. 2009. Web. <http://www.naturalnews.com/027691_hemp_protein_seeds.html>.

46. Wilcox, Julie. "7 Benefits Of Quinoa: The Supergrain Of The Future." *Forbes*. Forbes Magazine, 26 June 2012. Web. <http://www.forbes.com/sites/juliewilcox/2012/06/26/7-benefits-of-quinoa-the-supergrain-of-the-future/>.

47. "Quinoa." *The World's Healthiest Foods*. George Mateljan Foundation, n.d. Web. <http://www.whfoods.com/genpage.php?dbid=142>.

48. Jacoby, Christopher. "Health Benefits of Quinoa." *Health Guidance*. N.p., n.d. Web. <http://www.healthguidance.org/entry/14096/1/Health-Benefits-of-Quinoa.html>.

49. "Health Benefits of Quinoa." *Whole Grains Council*. N.p., n.d. Web. <http://www.wholegrainscouncil.org/whole-grains-101/health-benefits-of-quinoa>.

50. "Nutrition Facts." *And Analysis for Avocados, Raw, All Commercial Varieties*. N.p., n.d. Web. <http://nutritiondata.self.com/facts/fruits-and-fruit-juices/1843/2>.

51. "Power Foods: Lentils." *Whole Living*. N.p., Sept. 2006. Web. <http://www.wholeliving.com/133731/power-foods-lentils>.

52. Higdon, Jane, Ph.D. "Legumes." *Linus Pauling Institute*. Oregon State University, Dec. 2005. Web. <http://lpi.oregonstate.edu/infocenter/foods/legumes/>.

53. "Why Is It Important to Eat Grains, Especially Whole Grains?" *Choose My Plate*. USDA, n.d. Web. <http://www.choosemyplate.gov/food-groups/grains-why.html>.

54. "5 Health Benefits of Grains | Nutrition | Eat Well | Best Health." *Best Health*. N.p., n.d. Web. <http://www.besthealthmag.ca/eat-well/nutrition/5-health-benefits-of-grains>.

55. "Health Benefits of Grains." *Meals Matter Org*. N.p., n.d. Web. <http://www.mealsmatter.org/EatingForHealth/FunctionalFoods/Health-Benefits-of-Grains/>.

56. "Nutrition Facts." *And Analysis for Nuts, Almonds [Includes USDA Commodity Food A256, A264]*. N.p., n.d. Web. <http://nutritiondata.self.com/facts/nut-and-seed-products/3085/2>.

57. Brownlee, Iain, Andrew Fairclough, Anna Hall, and Jenny Paxman. *The Potential Health Benefits of Seaweed and Seaweed Extract*. Working paper. N.p.: n.p., n.d.*Sheffield Hallam University*. Web. <http://shura.shu.ac.uk/4980/1/The_Potential_Health_Benefits_of_Seaweed_and_Seaweed_Extracts.pdf>.

58. "Health Benefits of Seaweed." *Health Learning Info*. N.p., n.d. Web. <http://health.learninginfo.org/seaweed-benefits.htm>.

59. Trudeau, Kevin. *Natural Cures "they" Don't Want You to Know about.* Elk Grove Village, IL: Alliance Pub. Group, 2004. Print.

60. Young, Robert O. ., and Shelley Redford. Young. *The PH Miracle: Balance Your Diet, Reclaim Your Health.* New York: Grand Central Life & Style, 2010. Print.

61. Keenan, Susan M. "Pros And Cons Of Soy Milk." *Women's Health Issues.* N.p., 17 Sept. 2007. Web. 12 Dec. 2012. <http://www.lifescript.com/food/articles/p/pros_and_cons_of_soy_milk.aspx>.

62. "Pros and Cons of Drinking Soy Milk." *Fit Day.* N.p., n.d. Web. <http://www.fitday.com/fitness-articles/nutrition/healthy-eating/pros-and-cons-of-drinking-soy-milk.html>.

63. Barrera, Tatiana. "Love Your Health, Eat Alkaline Foods." *Eat Alkaline Foods.* N.p., 27 Oct. 2012. Web. <http://eatalkalinefoods.com/drinking-water>.

64. Batmanghelidj, F. Your Body's Many Cries for Water: You're Not Sick; You're Thirsty : Don't Treat Thirst with Medications. [Falls Church, VA]: Global Health Solutions, 2008. Print.

65. Batmanghelidj, F. Water: For Health, for Healing, for Life : You're Not Sick, You're Thirsty! New York: Grand Central Life & Style, 2012. Print.

66. Ozner, Michael D. Heart Attack Proof: A Six-week Cardiac Makeover for a Lifetime of Optimal Health. Dallas, TX: BenBella, 2012. Print.

67. Esselstyn, Rip. The Engine 2 Diet: The Texas Firefighter's 28-day Save-your-life Plan That Lowers Cholesterol and Burns Away the Pounds. New York: Wellness Central, 2009. Print.

68. Brian, Wendel, and John Corry, prods. "Forks Over Knives." *Forks Over Knives the Movie.* Dir. Lee Fulkerson. N.d. *Forks Over Knives.* Web. <http://www.forksoverknives.com/>.

69. Colquhoun, James, and Laurentine Ten Bosch, dirs. "Hungry for Change." *Hungry for Change the Movie.*

70. Colquhoun, James, and Laurentine Ten Bosch, dirs. "Food Matters" *Food Matters the Movie.*

71. Bedard, Megan. "100 Books on the Food Industry: If You Eat Food, Read Some."*TakePart.* N.p., 24 Mar. 2011. Web. <http://www.takepart.com/article/2011/03/24/100-books-food-industry-if-you-eat-food-read-some>.

72. Cross, Joe, and Kurt Engfehr, dirs. *Fat Sick and Nearly Dead | a Joe Cross Film.* N.d. Web. <http://www.fatsickandnearlydead.com/>.

73. Freston, Kathy. *Quantum Wellness*. London: Vermilion, 2008. Print.

74. Carr, Kris. Crazy Sexy Diet: Eat Your Veggies, Ignite Your Spark, and Live like You Mean It! Guilford, Ct: Skirt!, 2011. Print.

75. Freeman, Andrew, and Christina Kharbertyan. "18 'Food, Inc.' Facts Everyone Should Know." (n.d.): n. pag. *Take Part*. 24 Oct. 2012. Web. <http://www.takepart.com/photos/food-inc-facts/monsantos-soybean-monopoly>.

76. 13, December. "Cheese-making, Neolithic Style." *Los Angeles Times*. Los Angeles Times, 13 Dec. 2012. Web. <http://articles.latimes.com/2012/dec/13/science/la-sci-ancient-cheese-20121213>.

77. Reuters. "Humans Made Cheese 7,500 Years Ago." *MSN News*. N.p., 13 Dec. 2012. Web. <http://news.msn.com/science-technology/humans-made-cheese-7500-years-ago>.

78. Barrera, Tatiana. "Alkaline Food List." *Eat Alkaline Foods*. N.p., n.d. Web. <http://eatalkalinefoods.com/alkaline-foods-list/>.

www.ingramcontent.com/pod-product-compliance
Lightning Source LLC
Chambersburg PA
CBHW040128270326
41927CB00001B/22